LONGEVITY

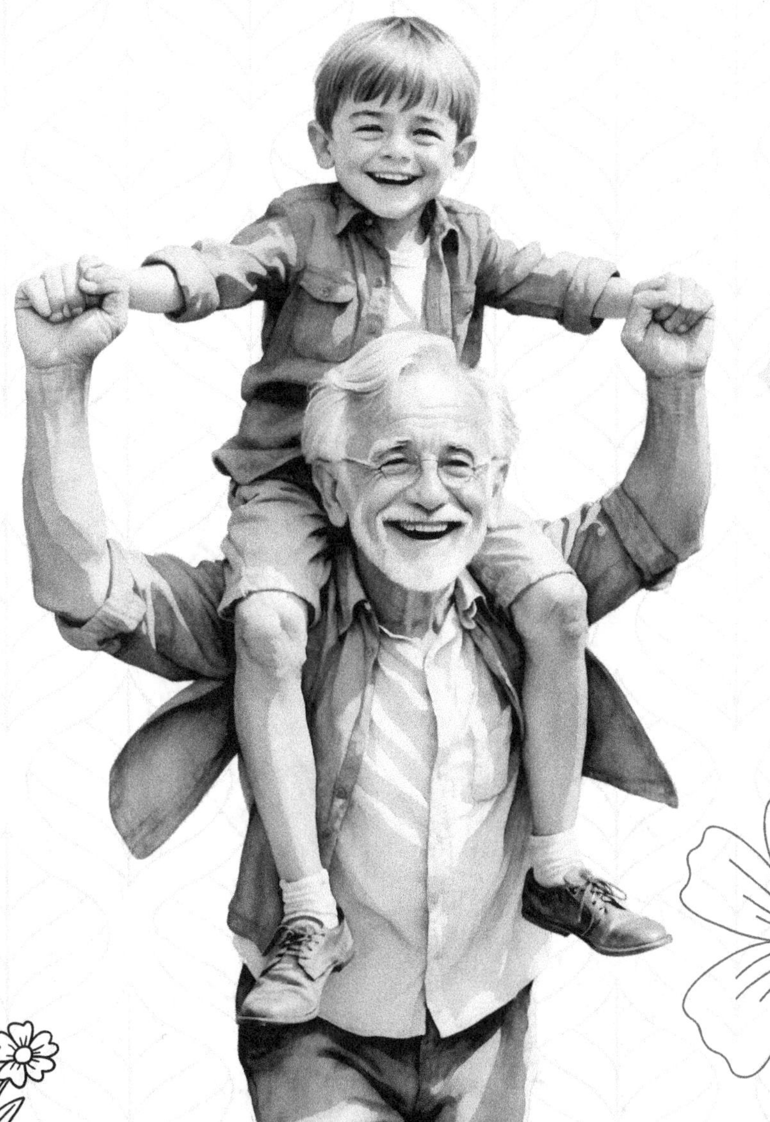

100 QUESTIONS
100 ANSWERS

100 Answers

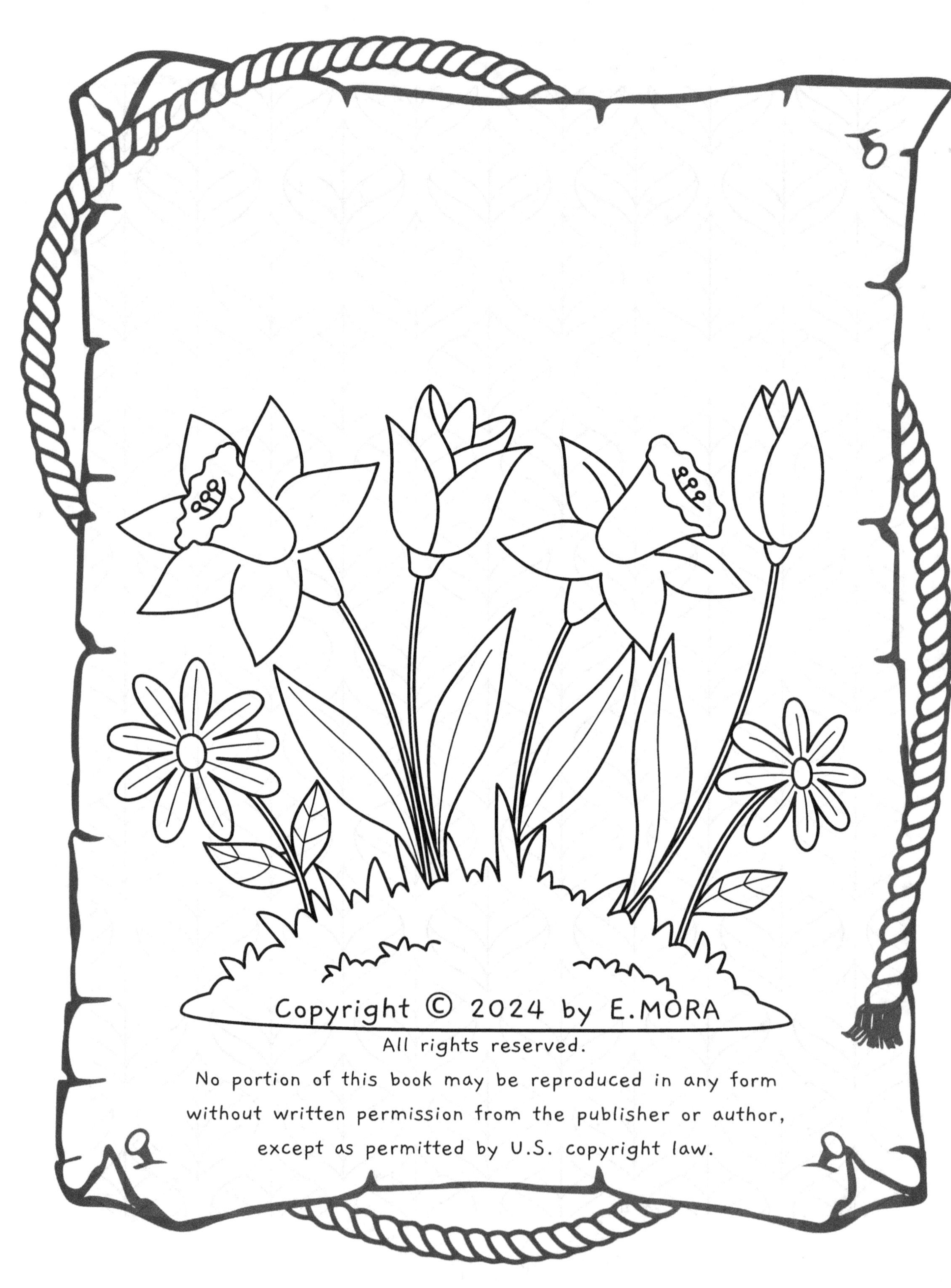

What is longevity?

Genetics, lifestyle choices, environmental factors, and access to healthcare all play roles in determining longevity.

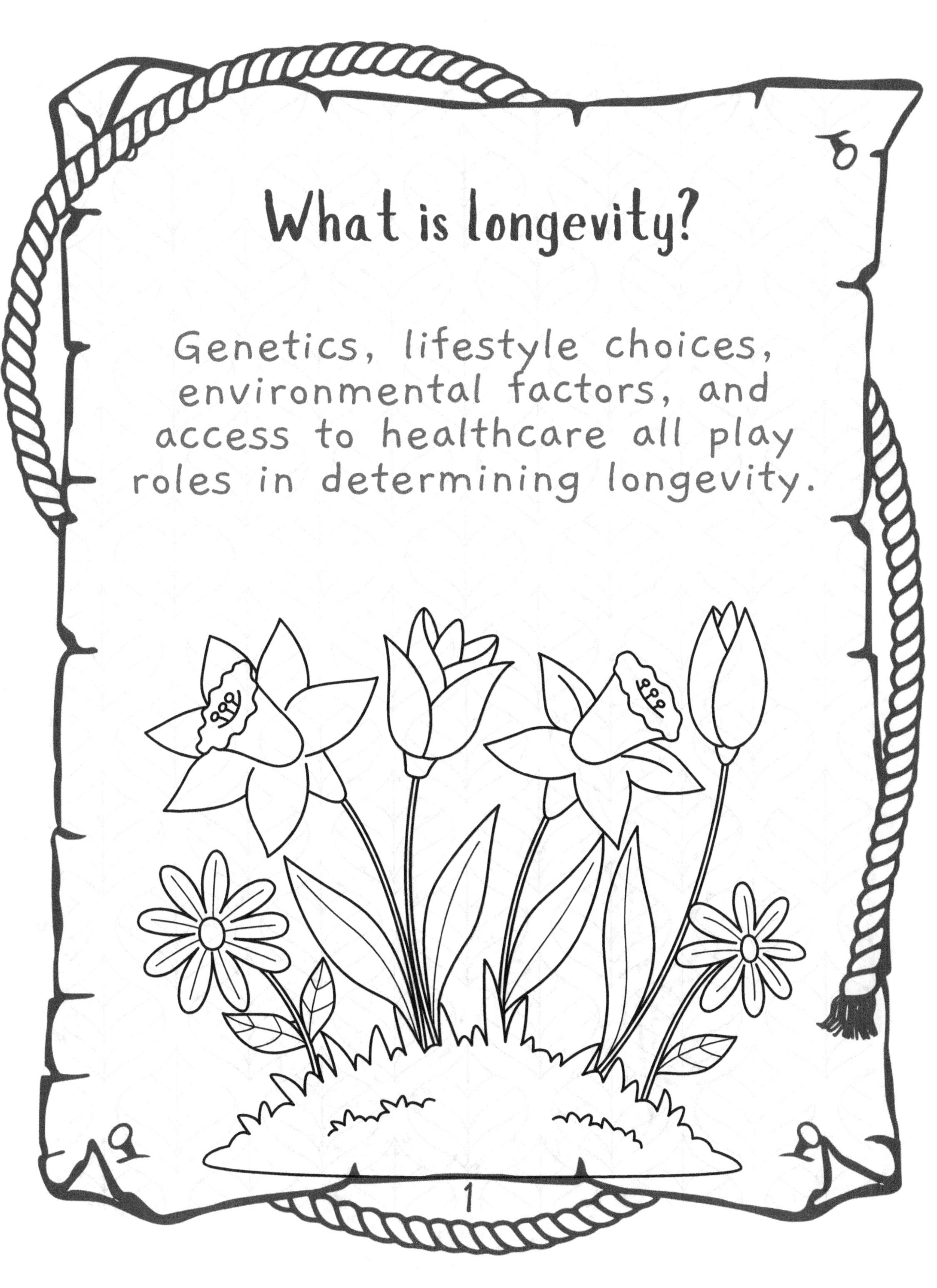

What factors contribute to longevity ?

Genetics, lifestyle choices, environmental factors, and access to healthcare all play roles in determining longevity.

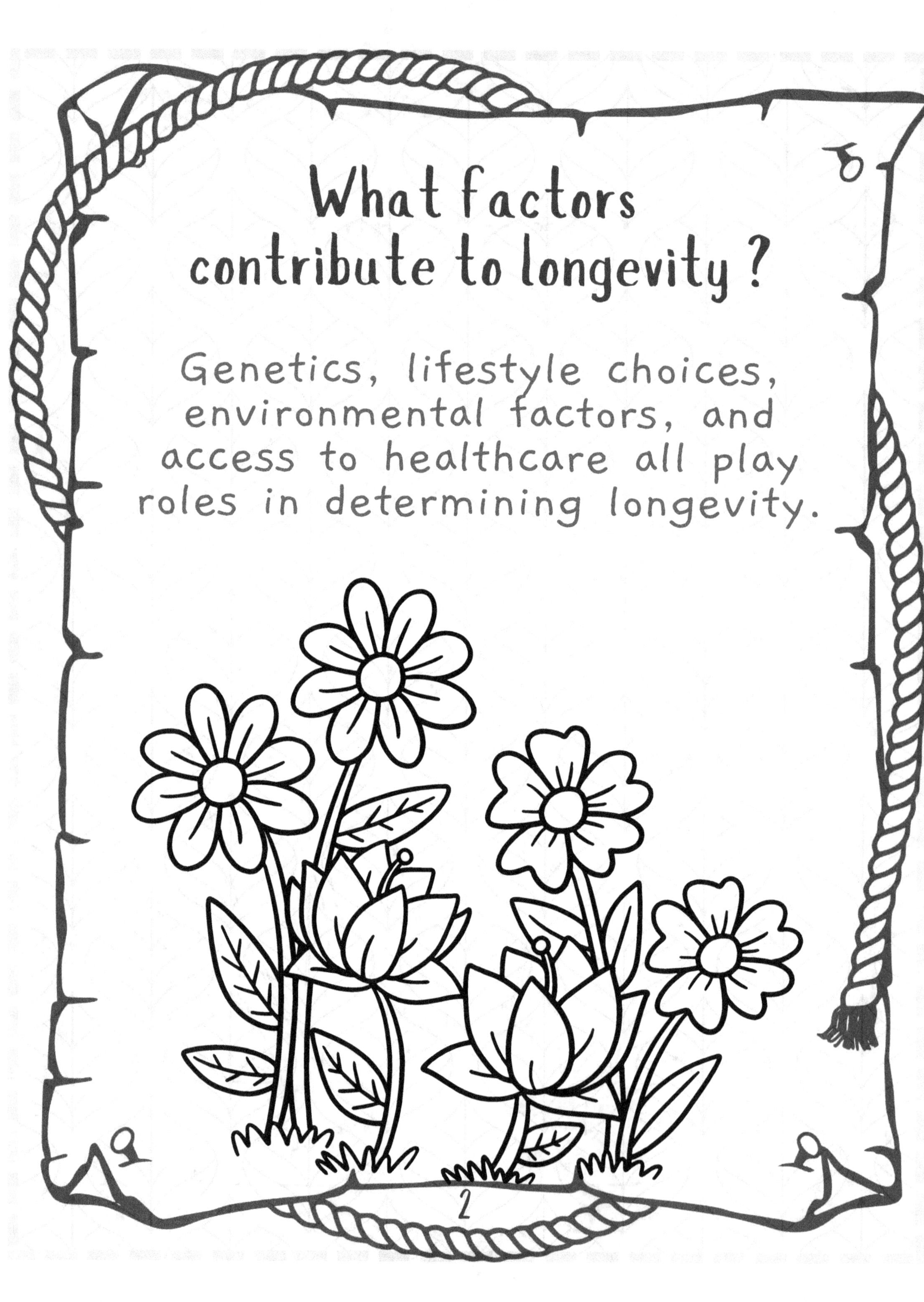

Can genetics influence how long someone lives?

Yes, genetics can influence longevity. Certain genes may predispose individuals to live longer or be more susceptible to specific health conditions.

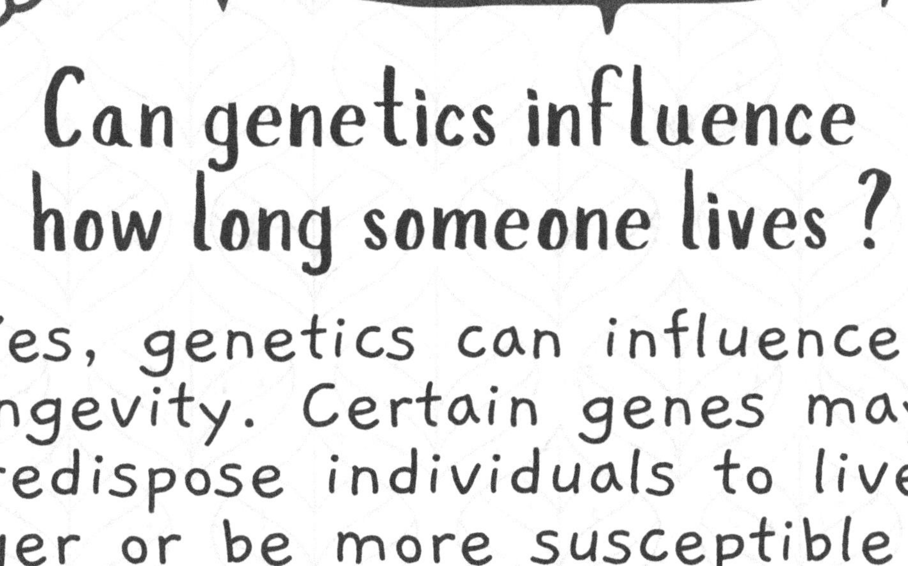

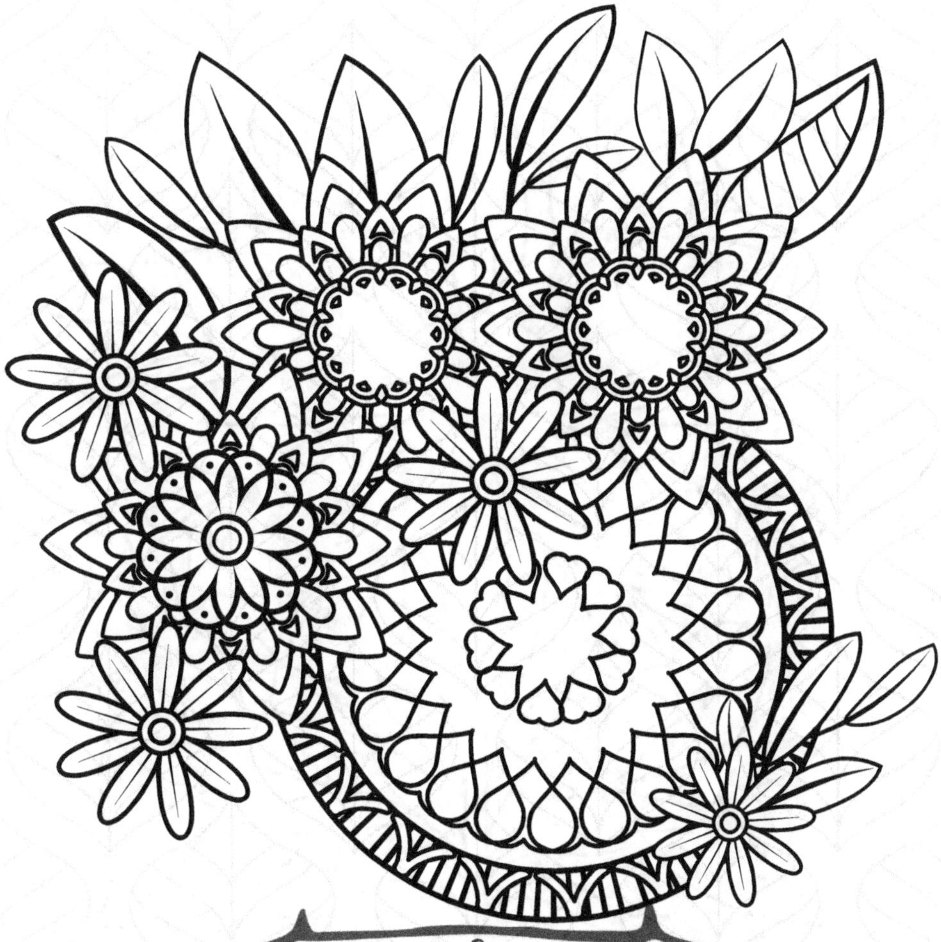

How does lifestyle impact longevity?

Healthy lifestyle choices such as regular exercise, balanced nutrition, and avoiding harmful habits like smoking can positively impact longevity.

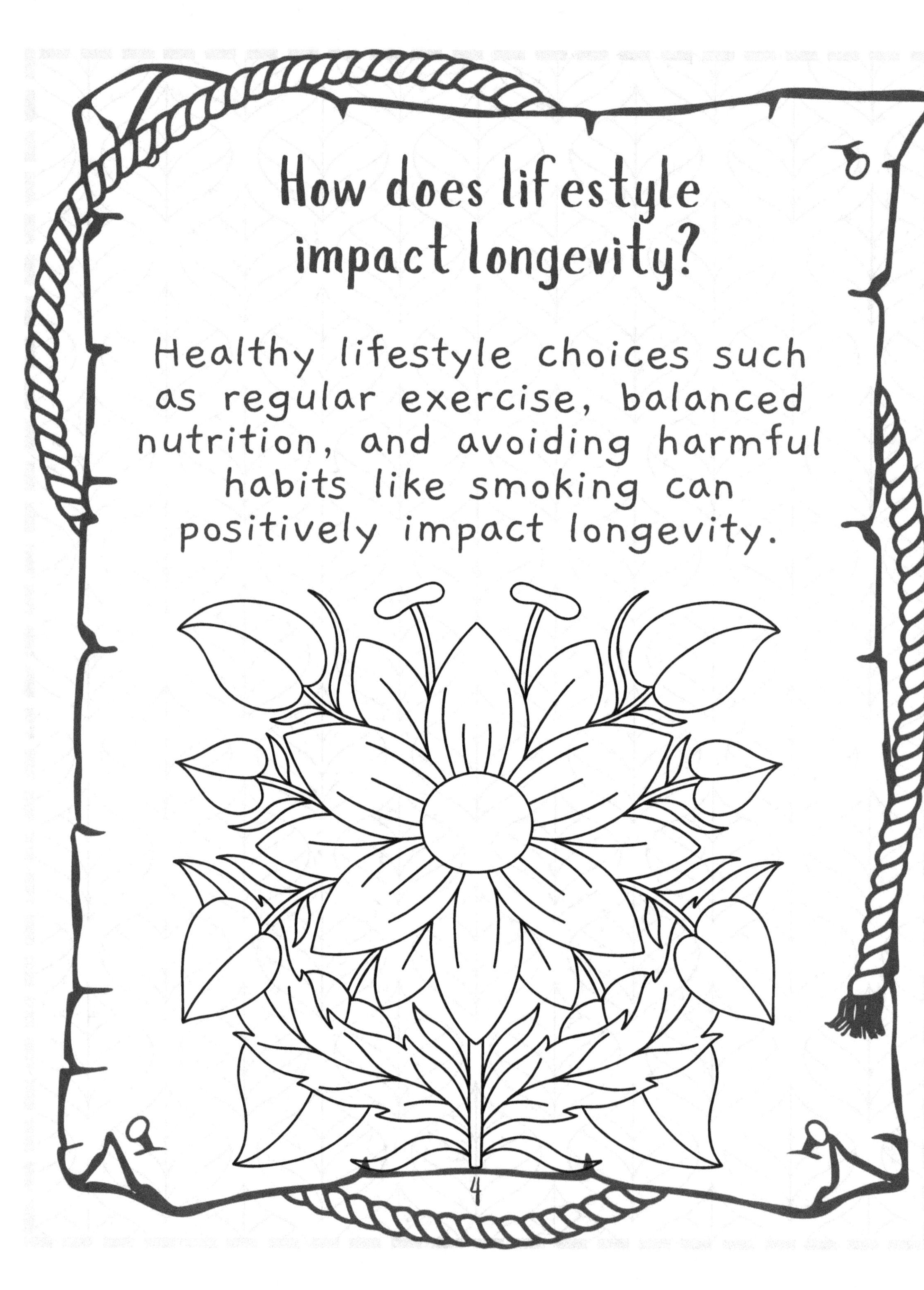

Are there specific diets linked to longevity?

Some diets, like the Mediterranean diet, have been associated with increased longevity due to their focus on whole foods, lean proteins, and healthy fats.

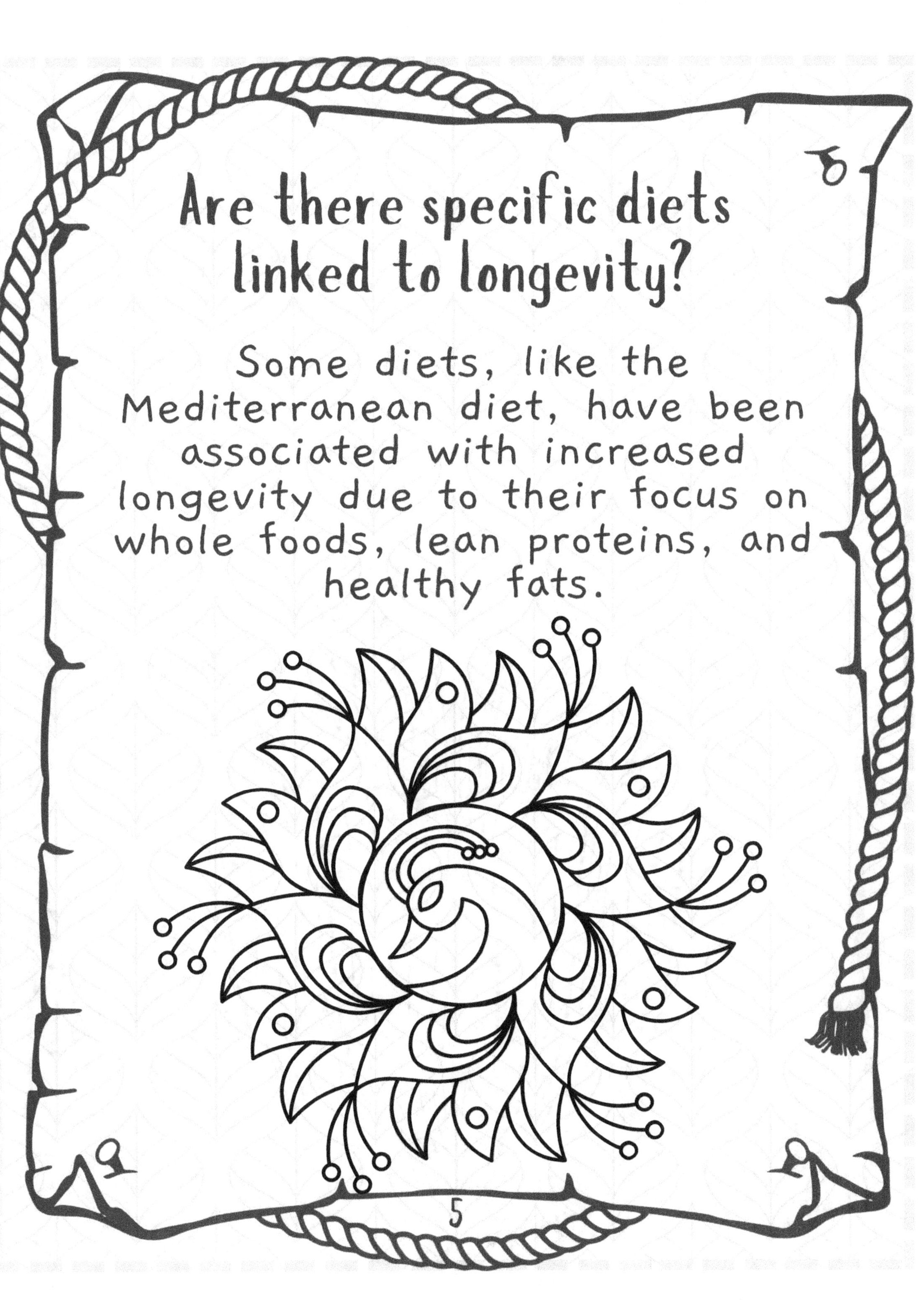

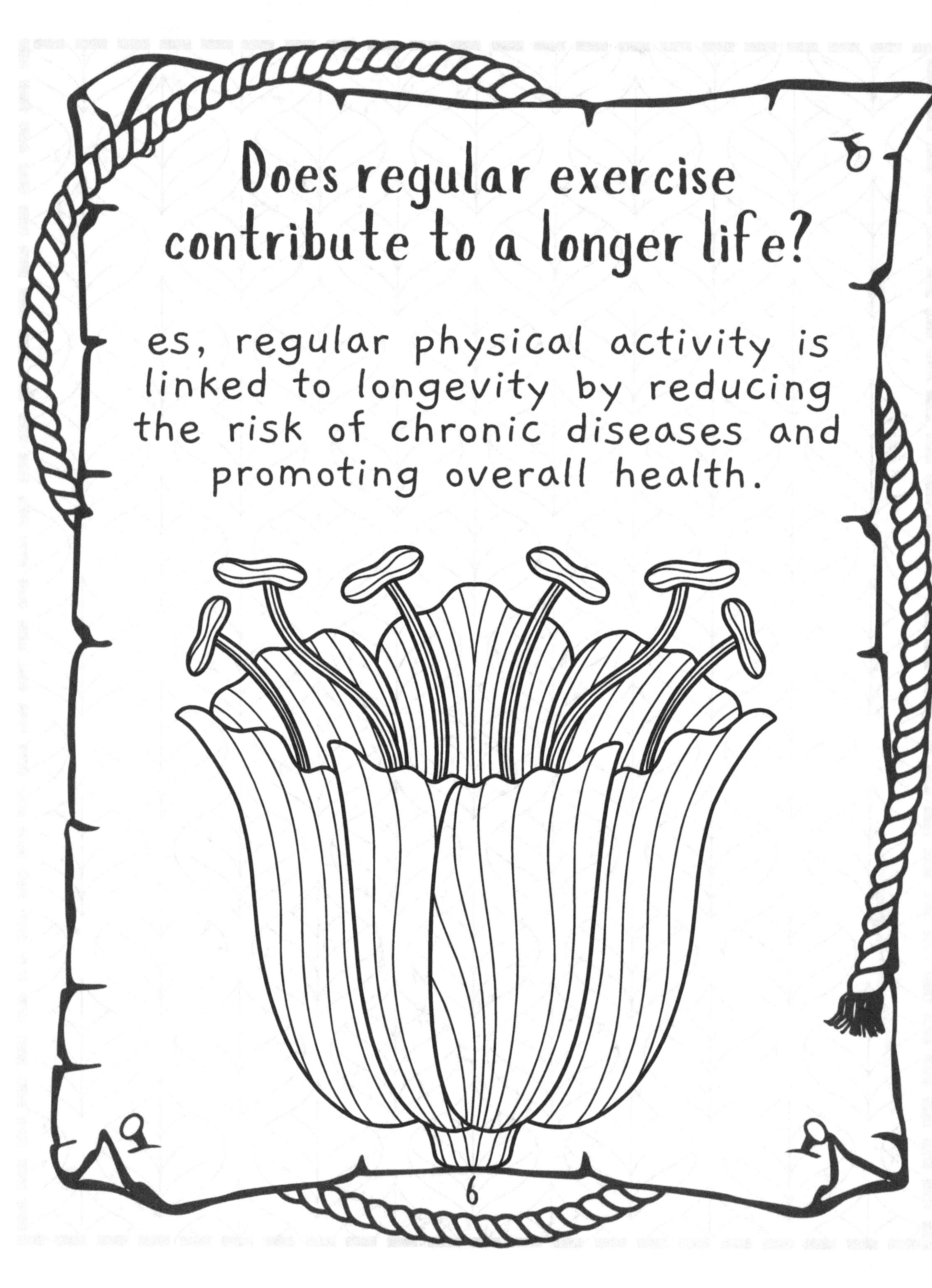

Does regular exercise contribute to a longer life?

es, regular physical activity is linked to longevity by reducing the risk of chronic diseases and promoting overall health.

Can social connections influence longevity?

Yes, strong social connections and a supportive social network have been linked to increased lifespan.

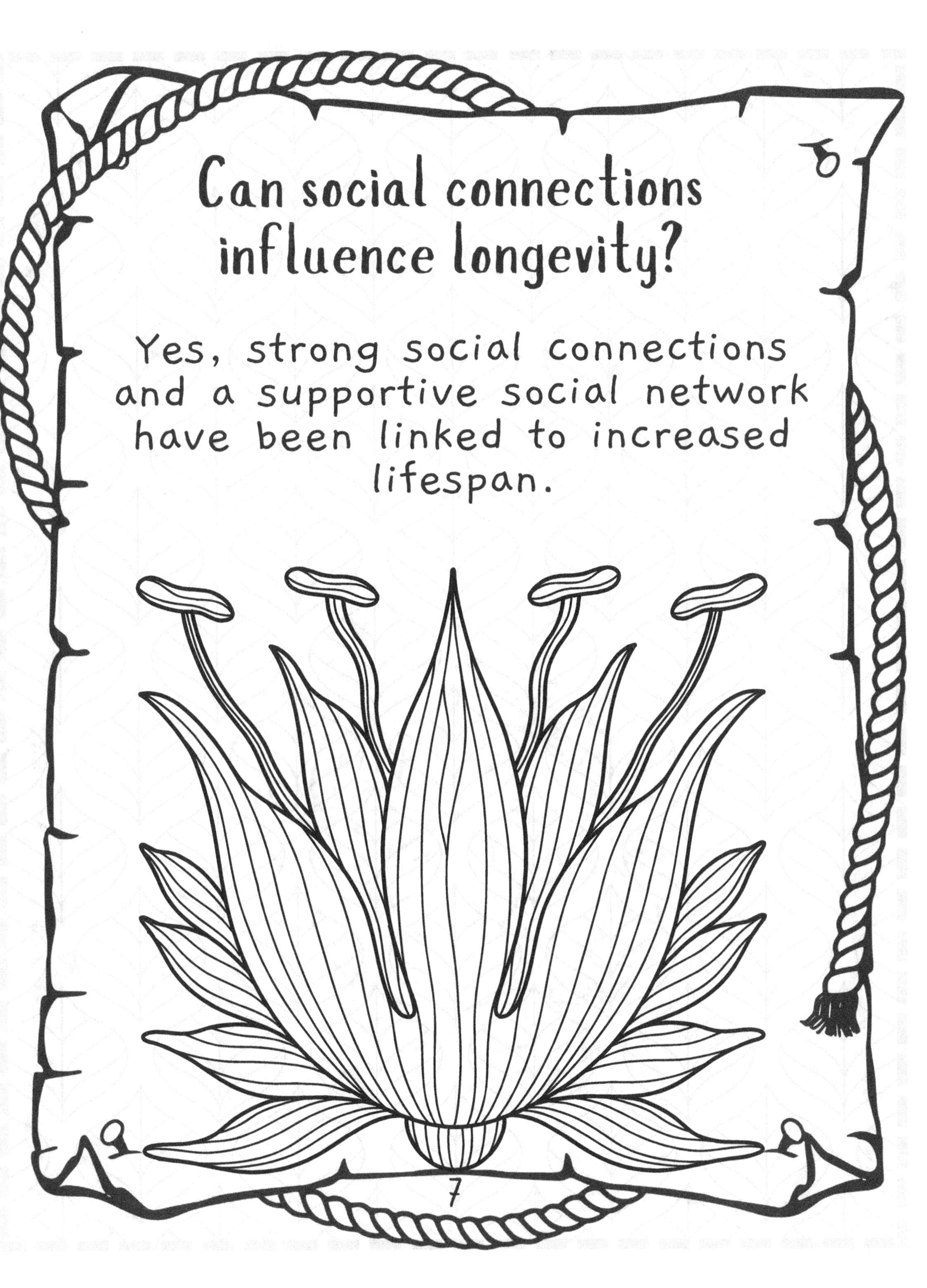

How does stress affect longevity?

Chronic stress can negatively impact health and potentially shorten lifespan. Managing stress is crucial for promoting longevity.

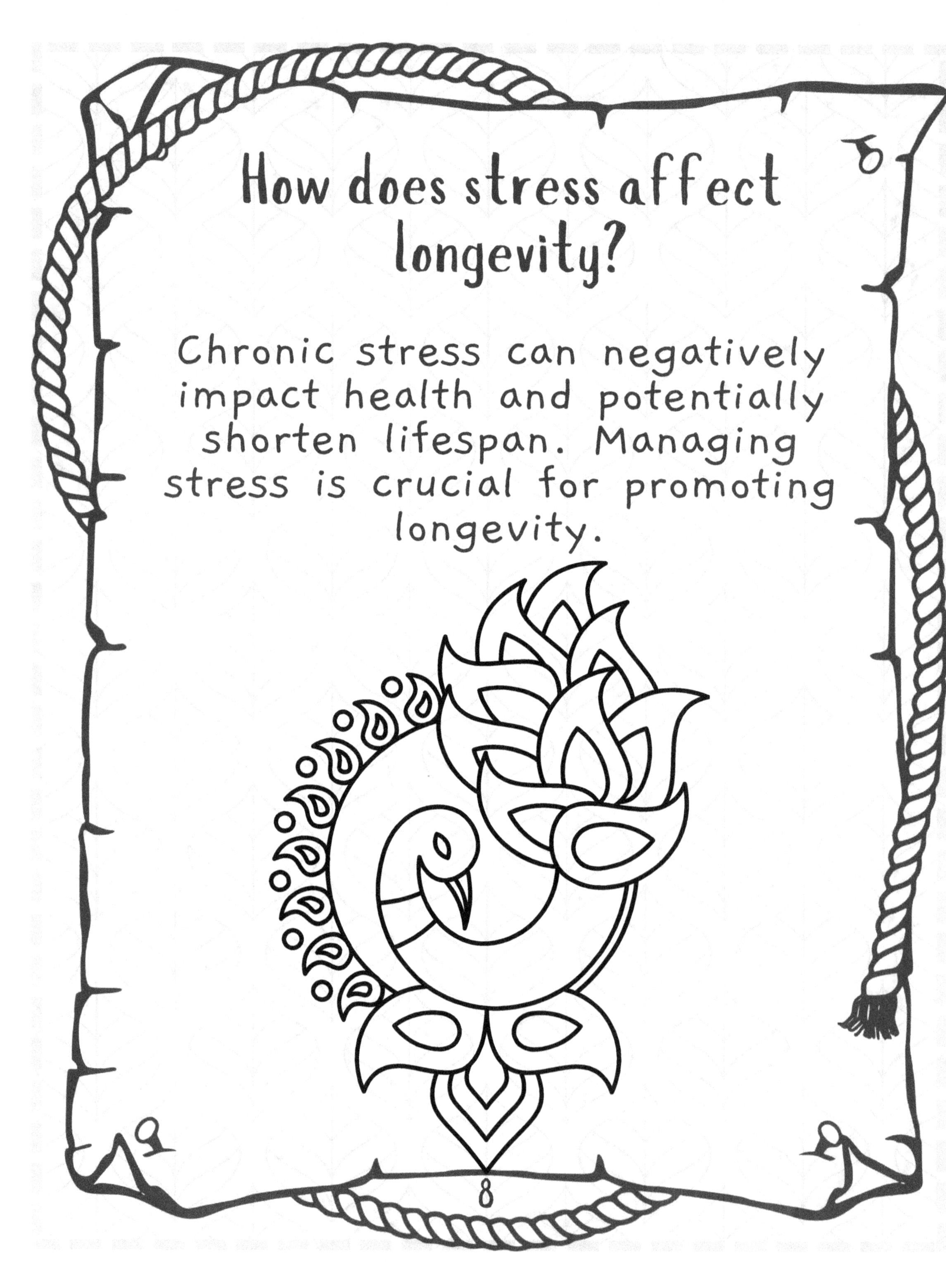

Is there a relationship between sleep and longevity?

Yes, adequate and quality sleep is essential for overall health and has been associated with increased longevity.

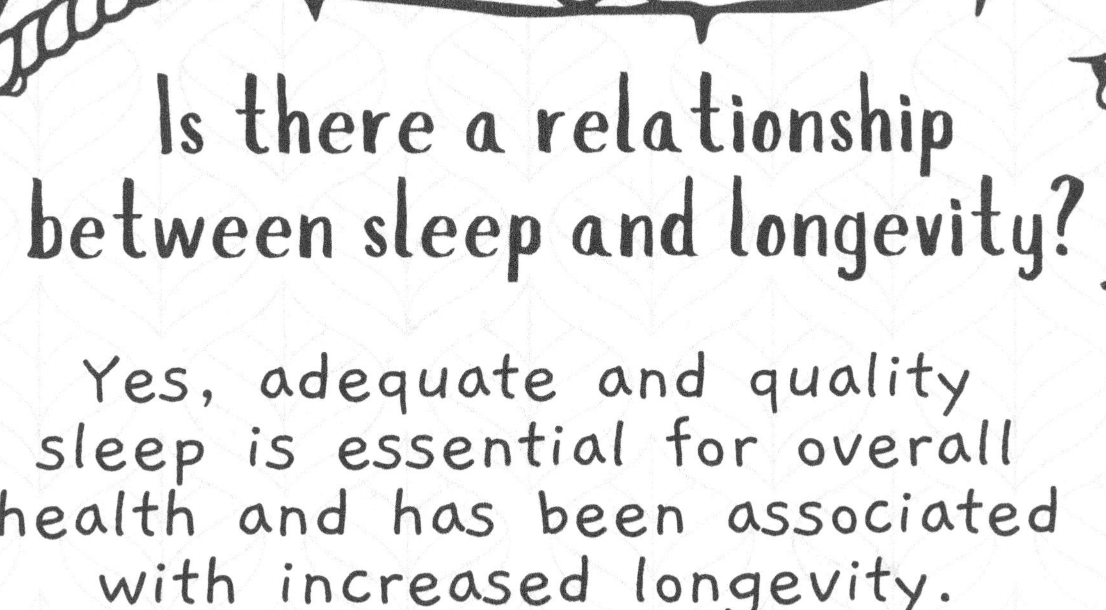

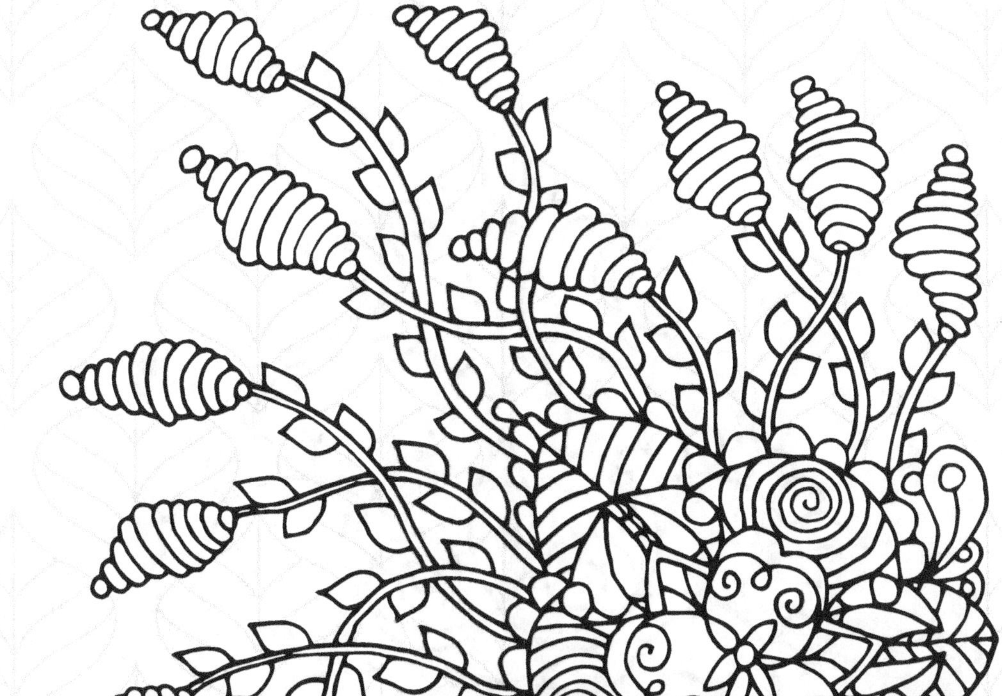

Can advances in medical technology contribute to increased longevity?

Medical advancements, such as improved treatments and early disease detection, can contribute to increased longevity.

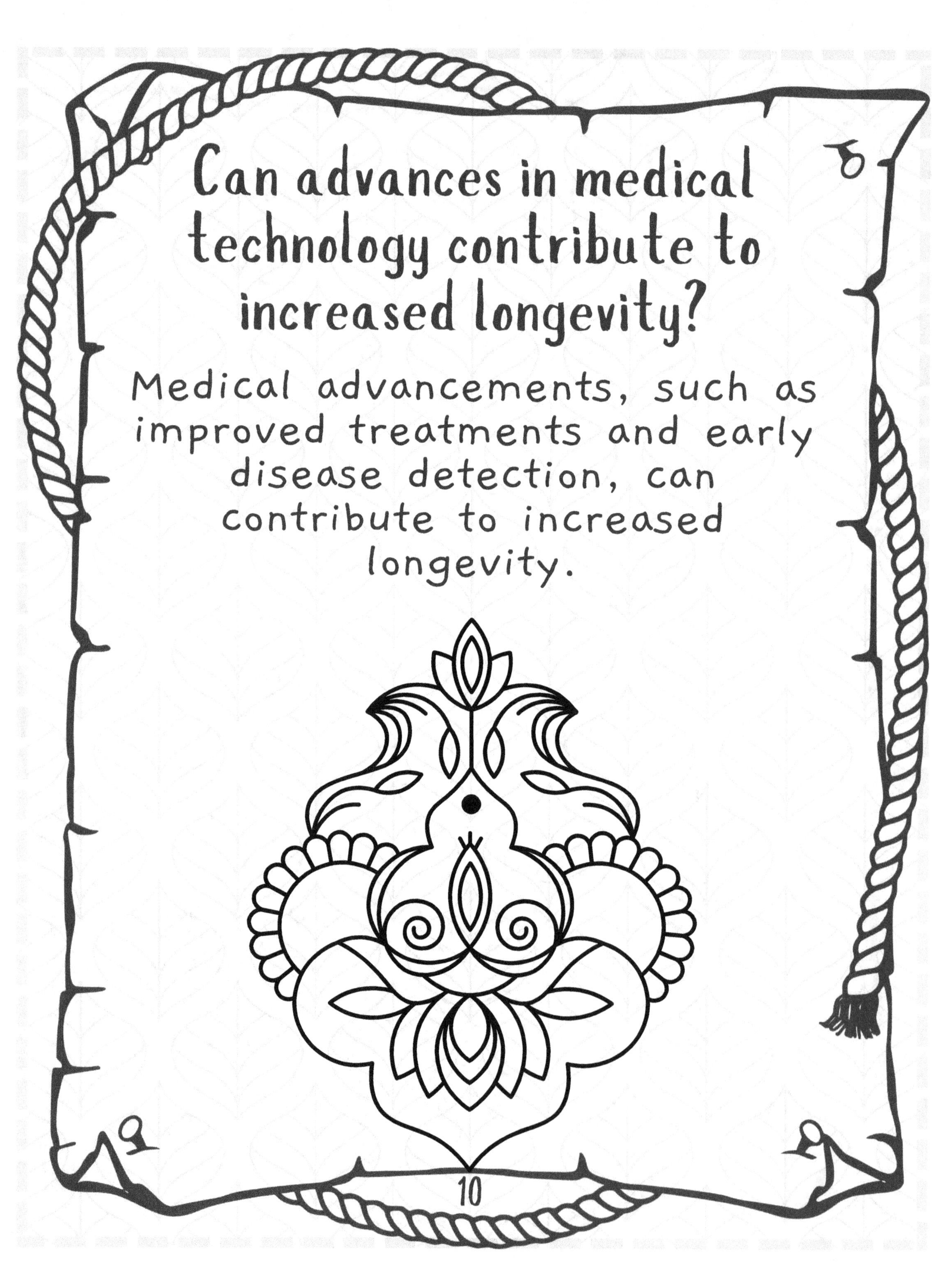

Are there specific anti-aging treatments available?

While no definitive anti-aging treatments exist, certain lifestyle choices and some medical interventions may slow down the aging process.

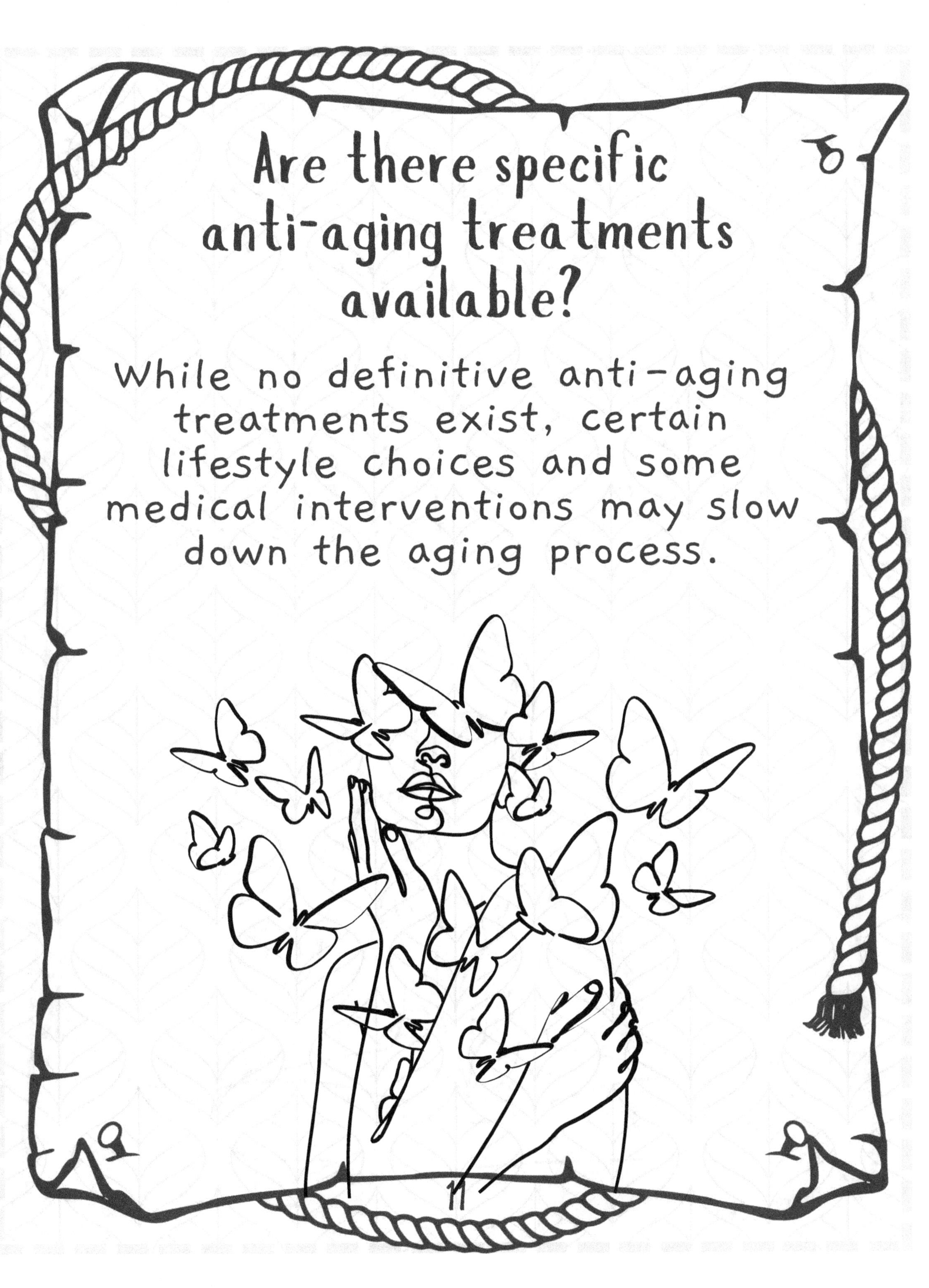

How does calorie restriction impact longevity?

Calorie restriction has been studied for its potential to extend lifespan by promoting metabolic health, although more research is needed.

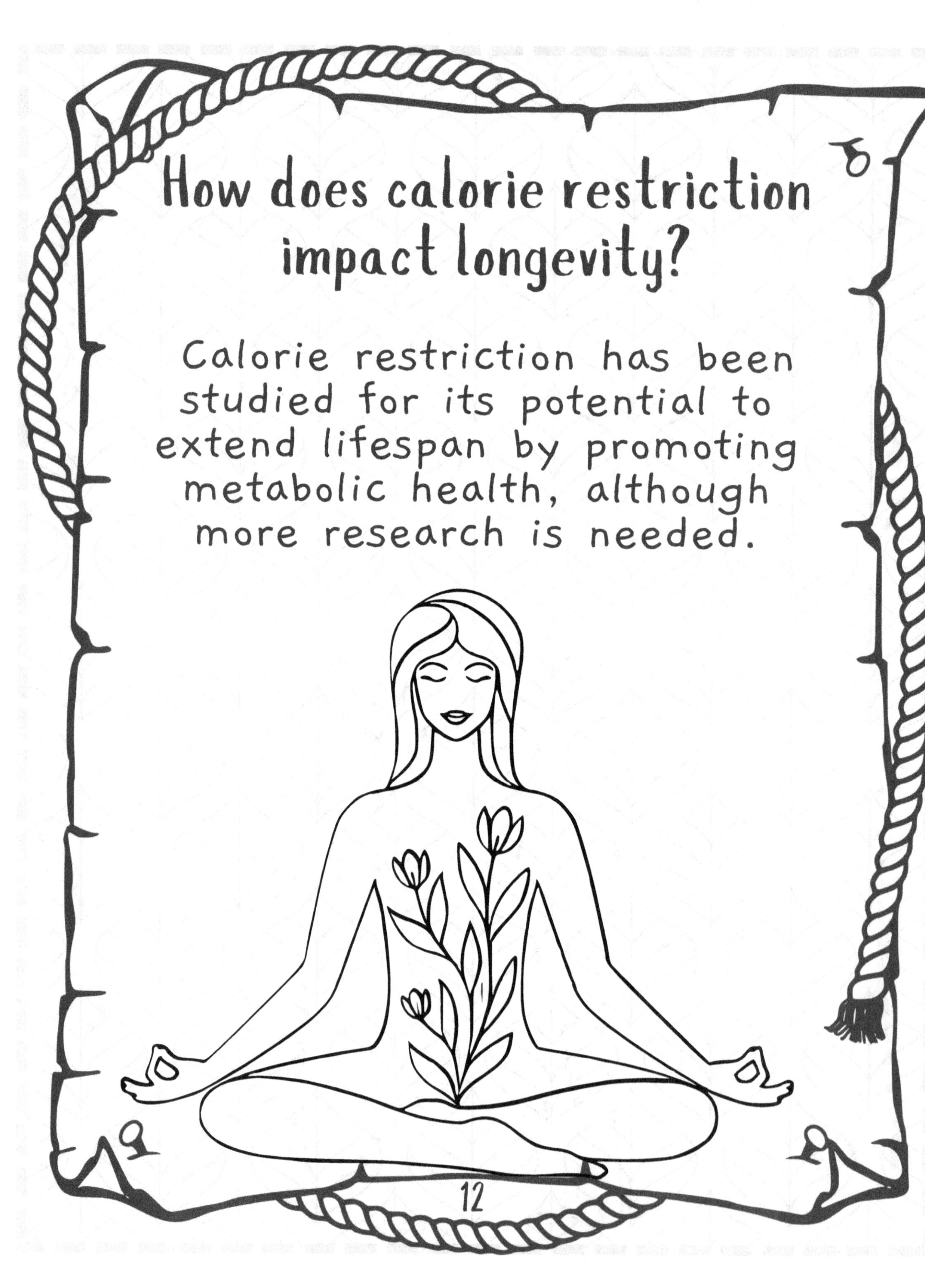

Can genetic engineering play a role in extending human lifespan?

Some research explores genetic interventions to slow aging, but ethical and safety considerations make this area complex.

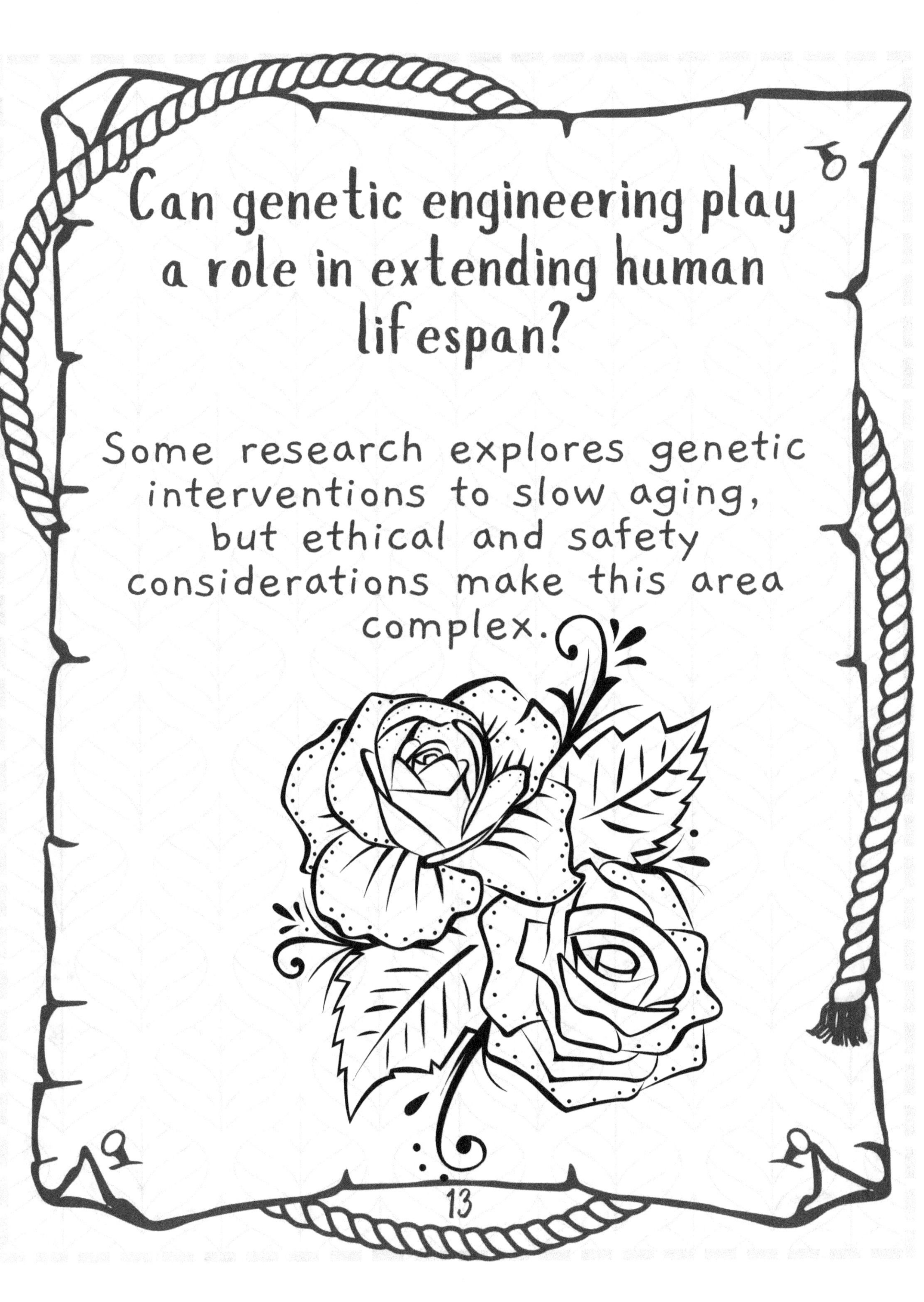

What role do antioxidants play in longevity?

Antioxidants may help combat oxidative stress, potentially influencing longevity, but the relationship is not fully understood.

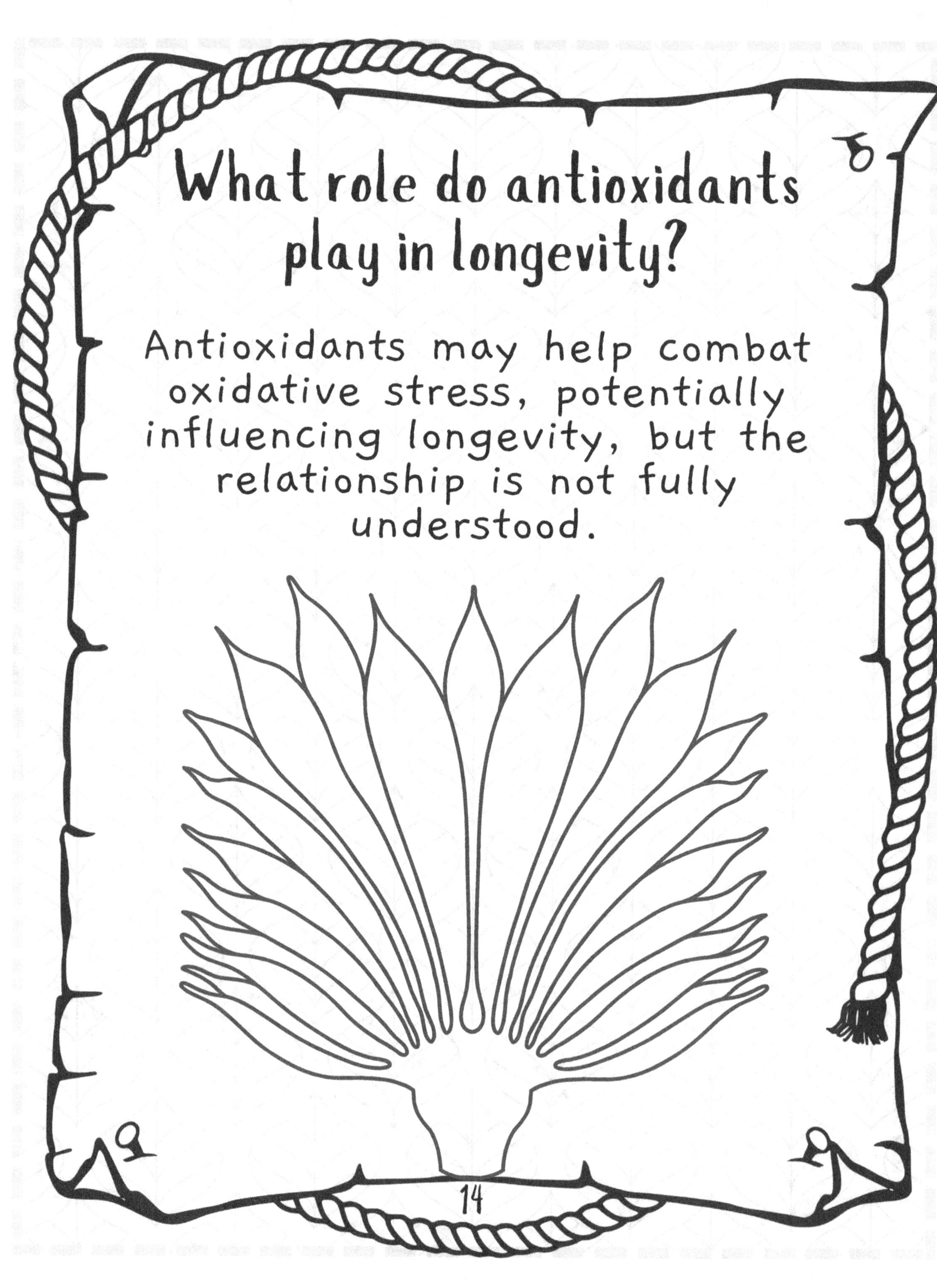

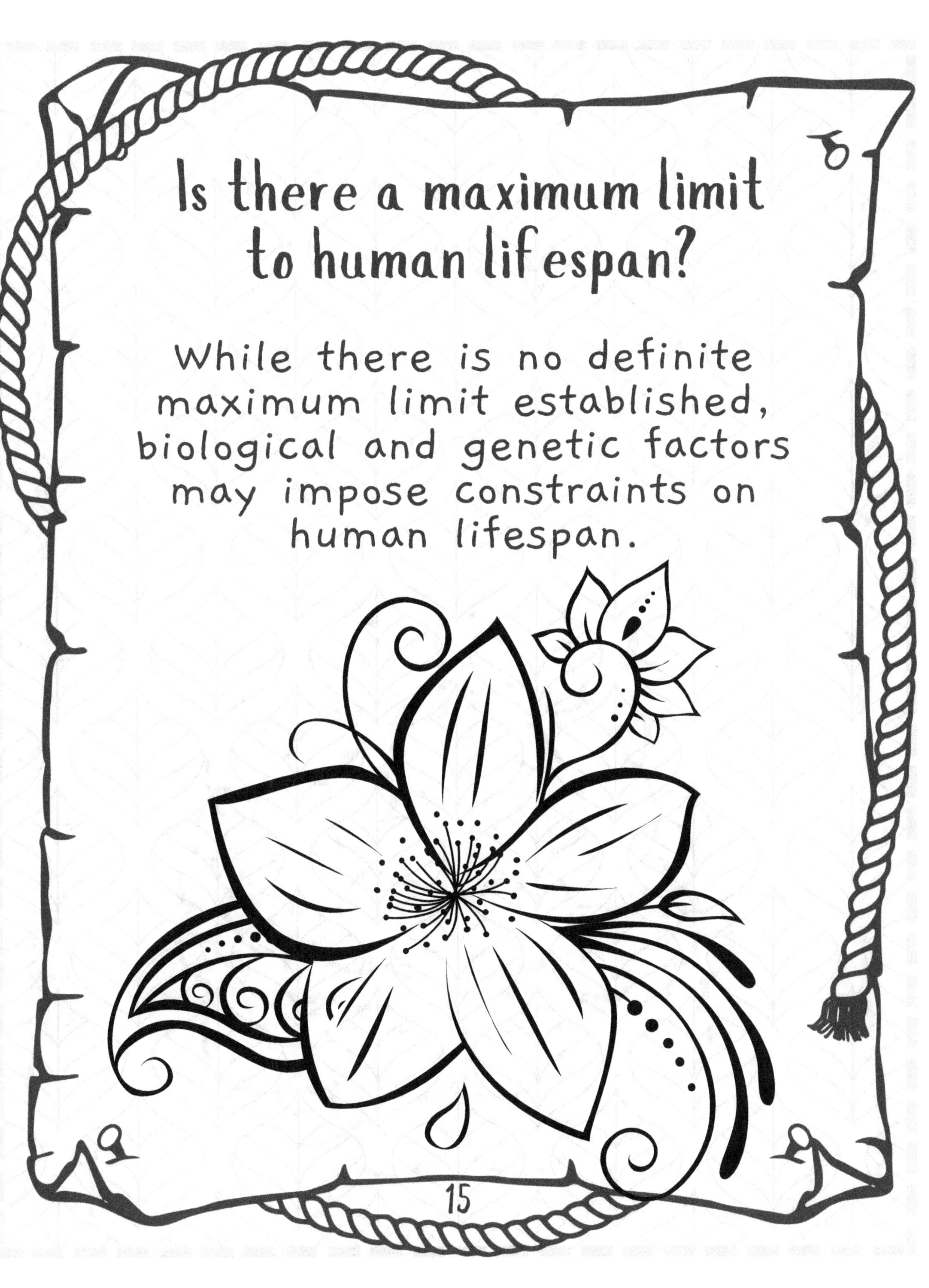

Is there a maximum limit
to human lifespan?

While there is no definite
maximum limit established,
biological and genetic factors
may impose constraints on
human lifespan.

Can mental health influence how long someone lives?

Mental health is connected to overall well-being, and positive mental health can contribute to increased longevity.

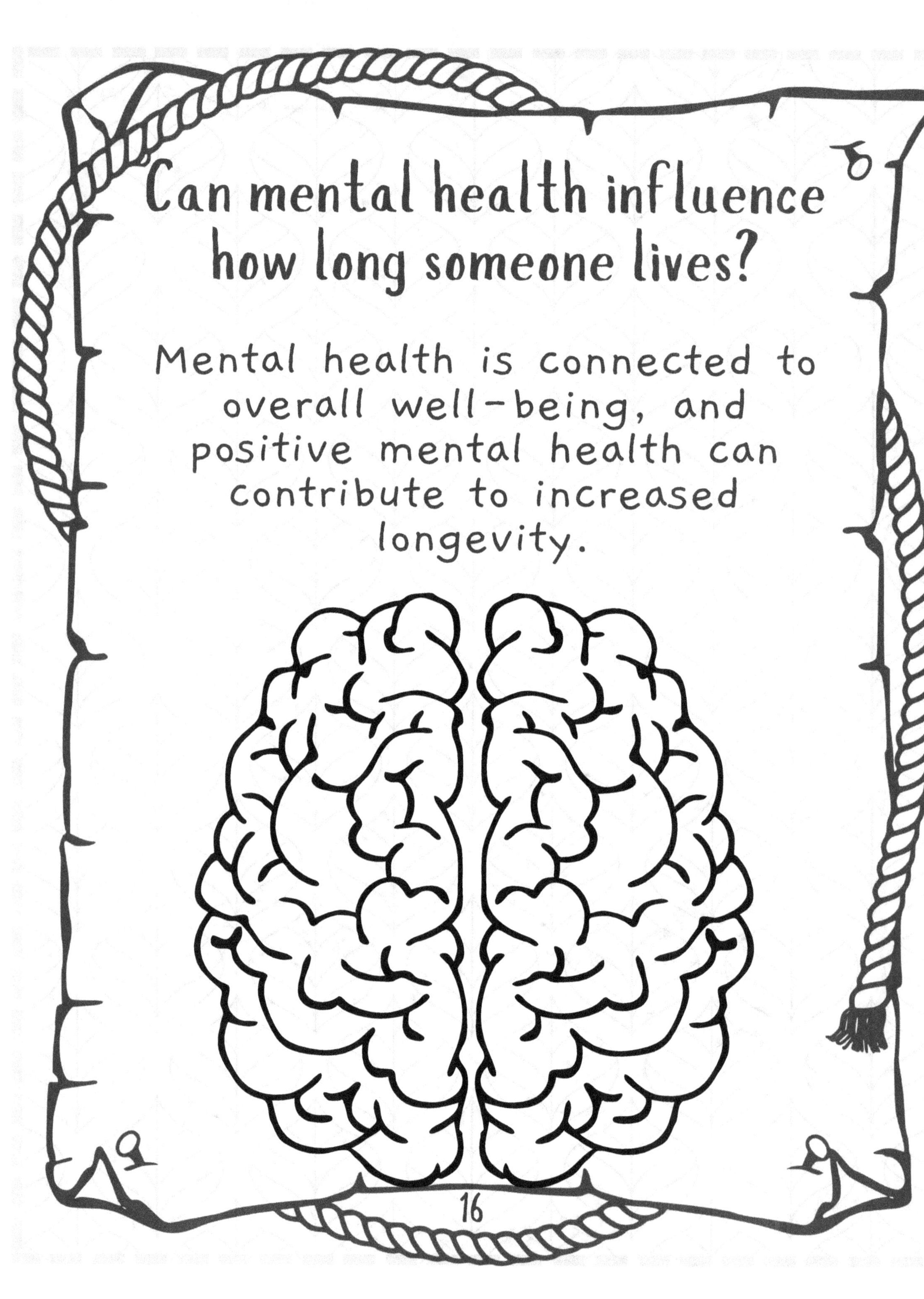

How does environmental pollution impact longevity?

Prolonged exposure to environmental pollutants can have adverse health effects, potentially impacting longevity.

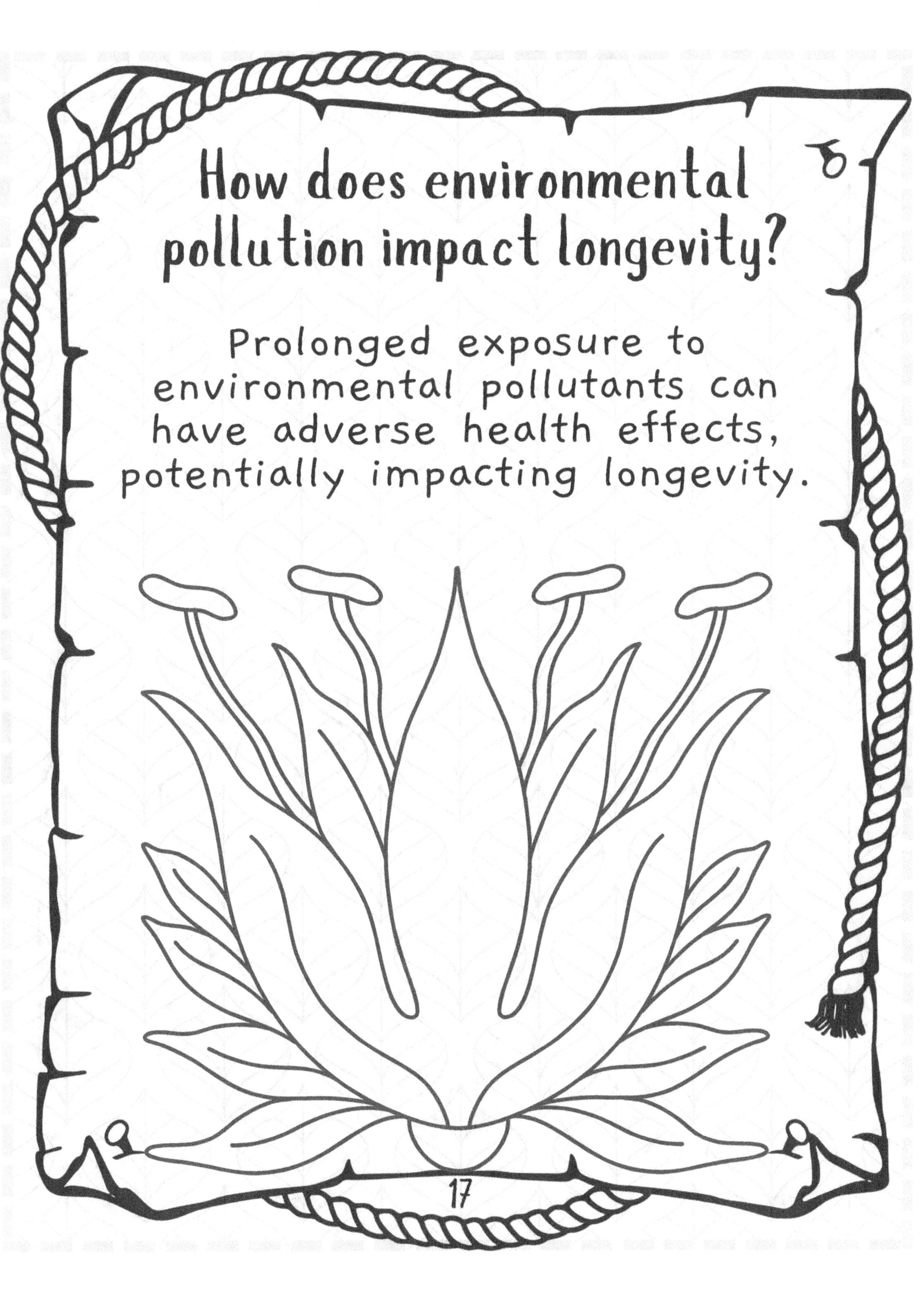

Are there specific regions with higher longevity rates?

Certain regions, like the "Blue Zones," have been identified where people tend to live longer, often attributed to lifestyle and diet.

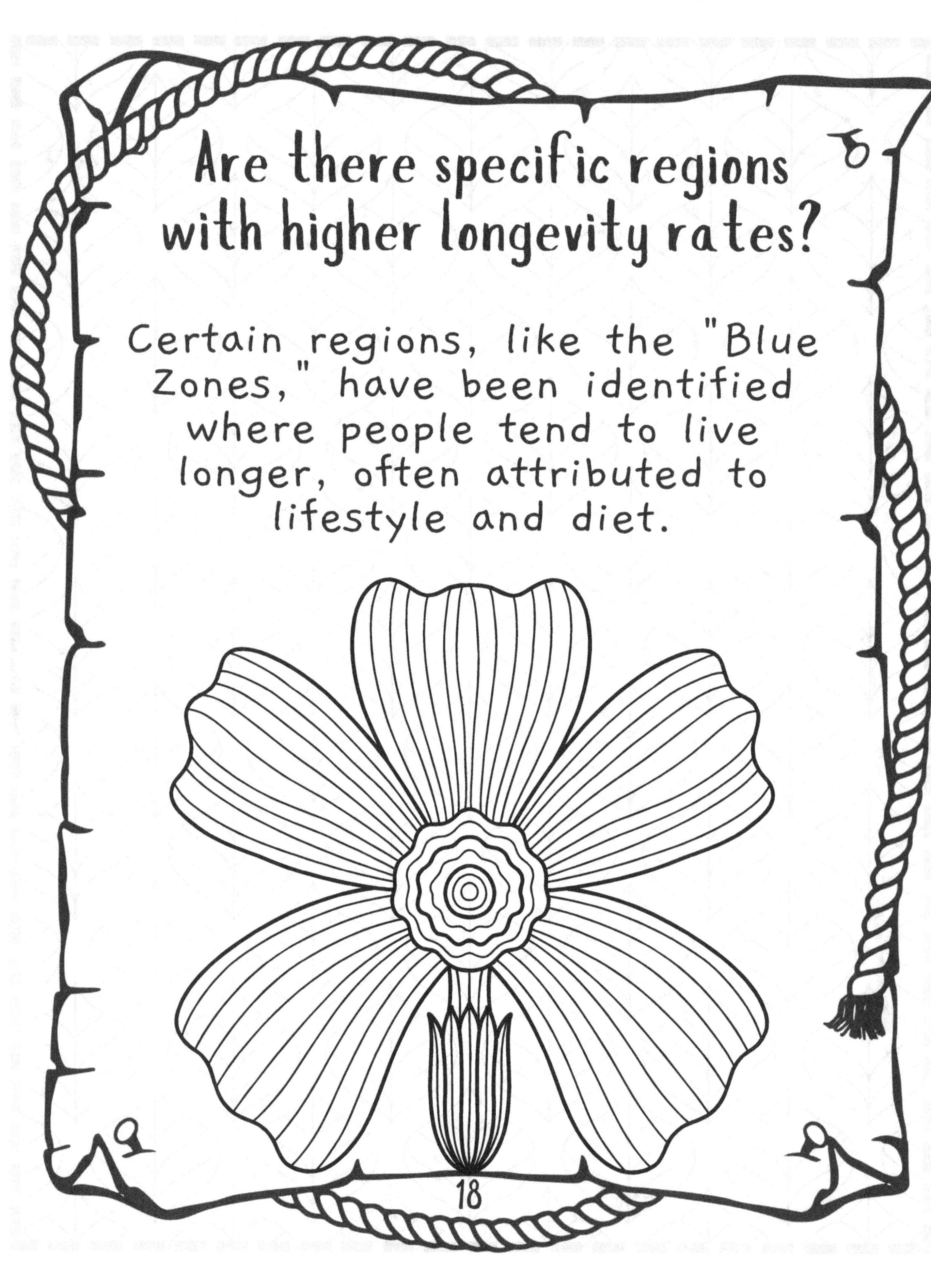

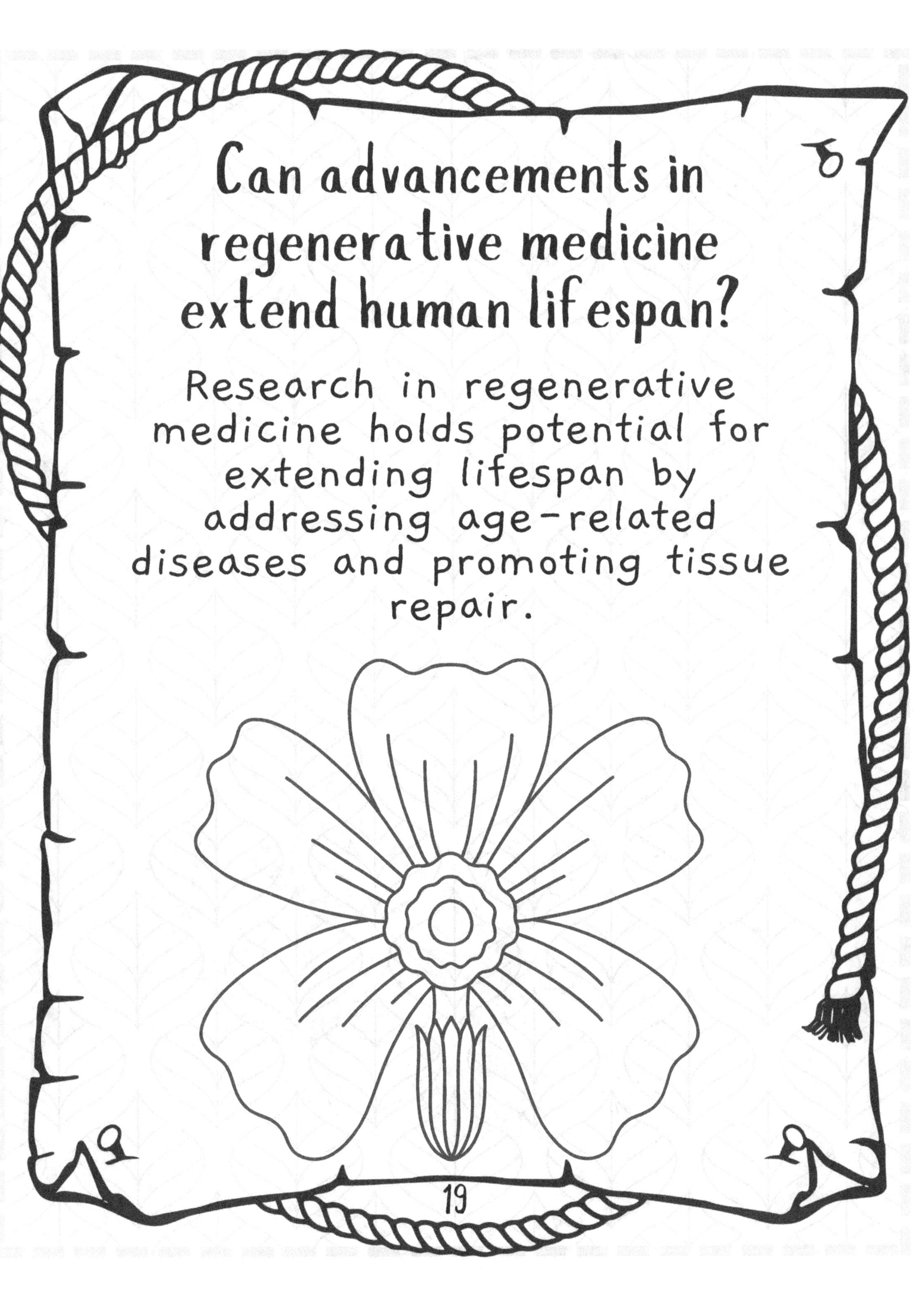

Can advancements in regenerative medicine extend human lifespan?

Research in regenerative medicine holds potential for extending lifespan by addressing age-related diseases and promoting tissue repair.

What is the role of genetics in personalized longevity interventions?

Personalized interventions based on genetic information may become more prevalent, tailoring approaches to an individual's unique genetic makeup for optimal health and longevity.

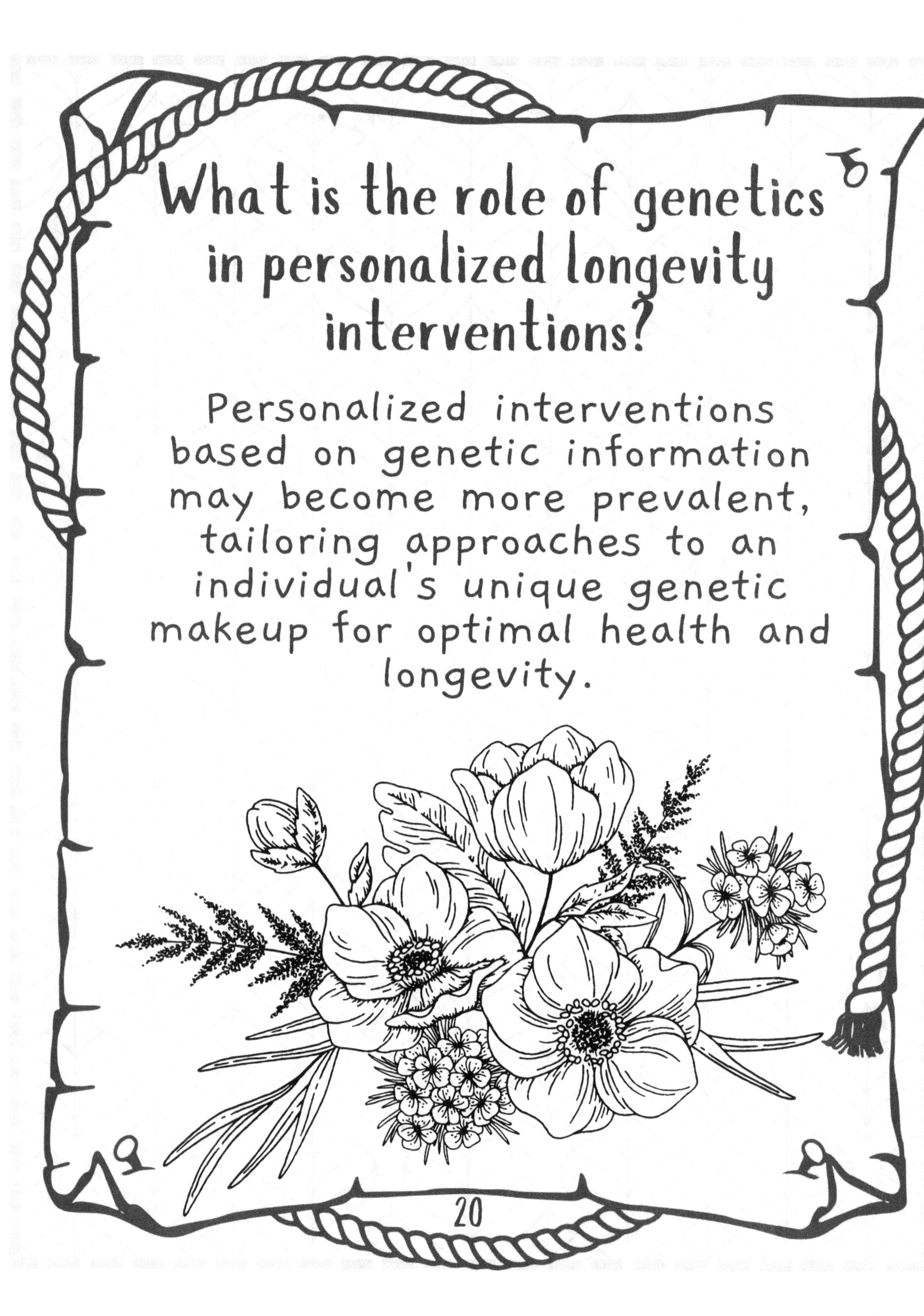

Can the study of telomeres provide insights into longevity?

Telomeres, the protective caps at the end of chromosomes, are associated with cellular aging. Research suggests that maintaining telomere length may play a role in promoting longevity.

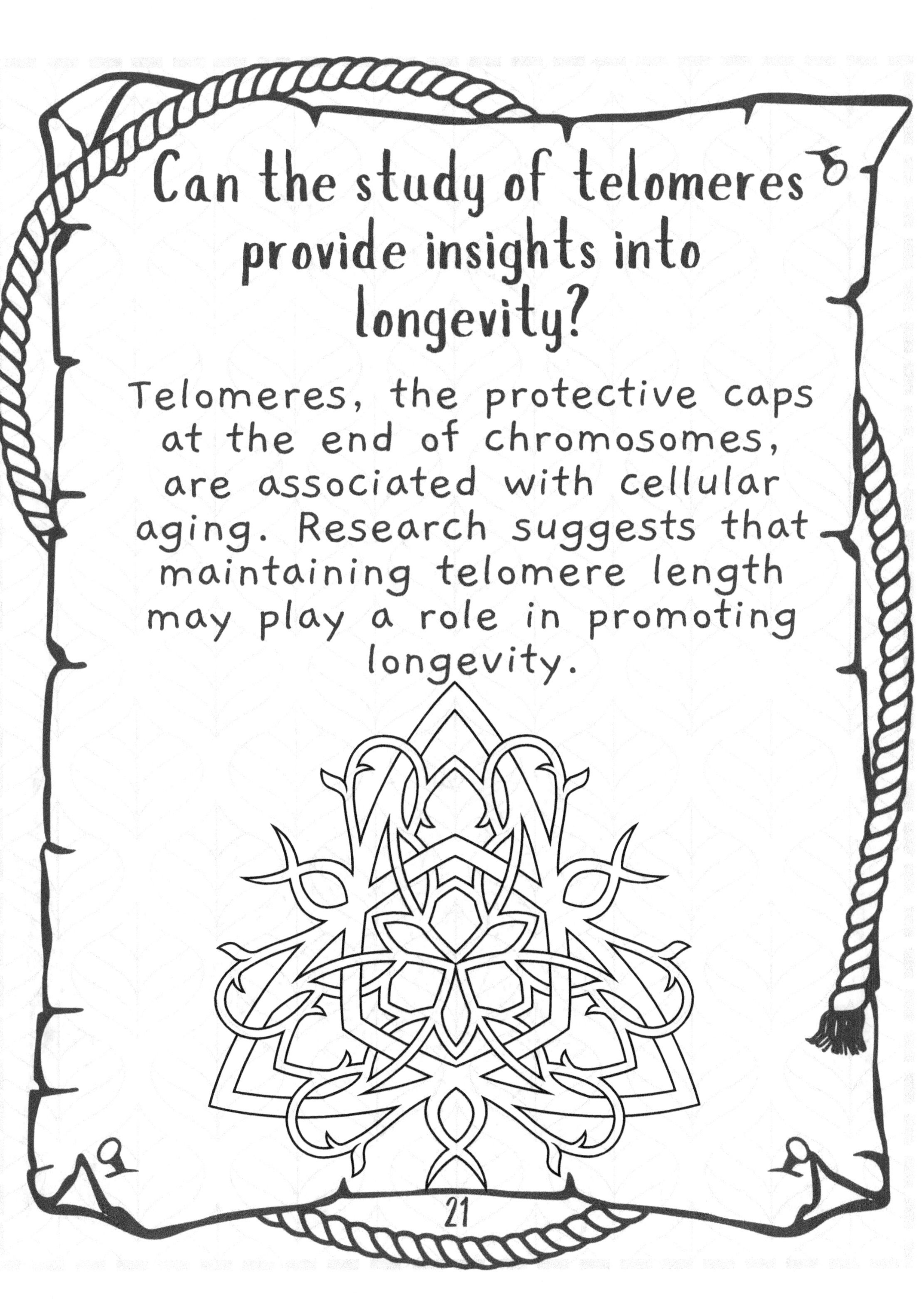

How does the gut microbiome impact longevity?

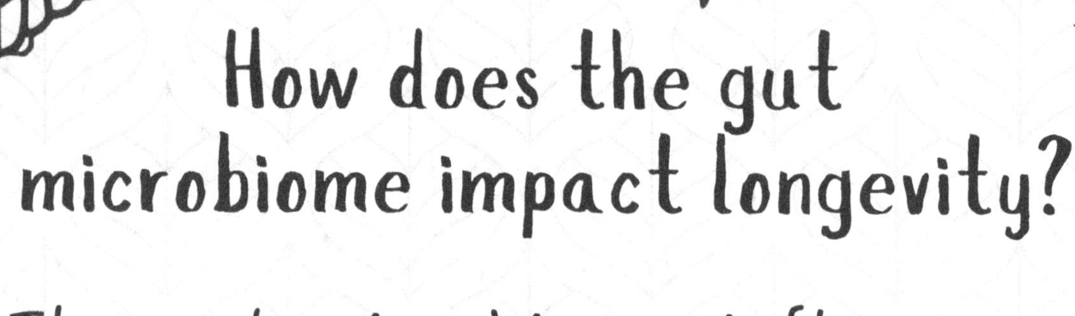

The gut microbiome influences various aspects of health, and emerging research suggests a connection between a balanced gut microbiota and increased lifespan.

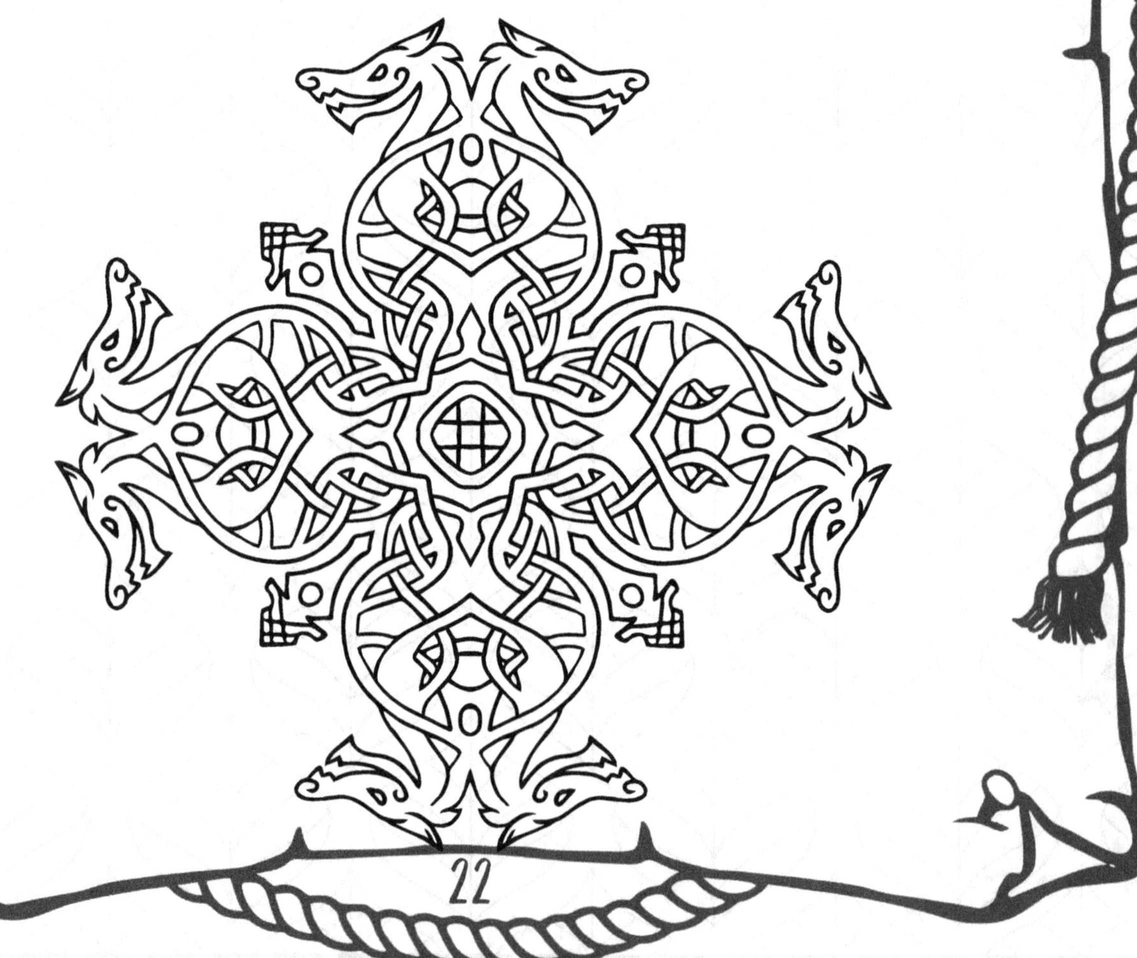

Are there any lifestyle practices from centenarians that promote longevity?

Centenarians in certain cultures often share lifestyle practices such as a strong sense of community, plant-based diets, and staying physically active, which may contribute to their longevity.

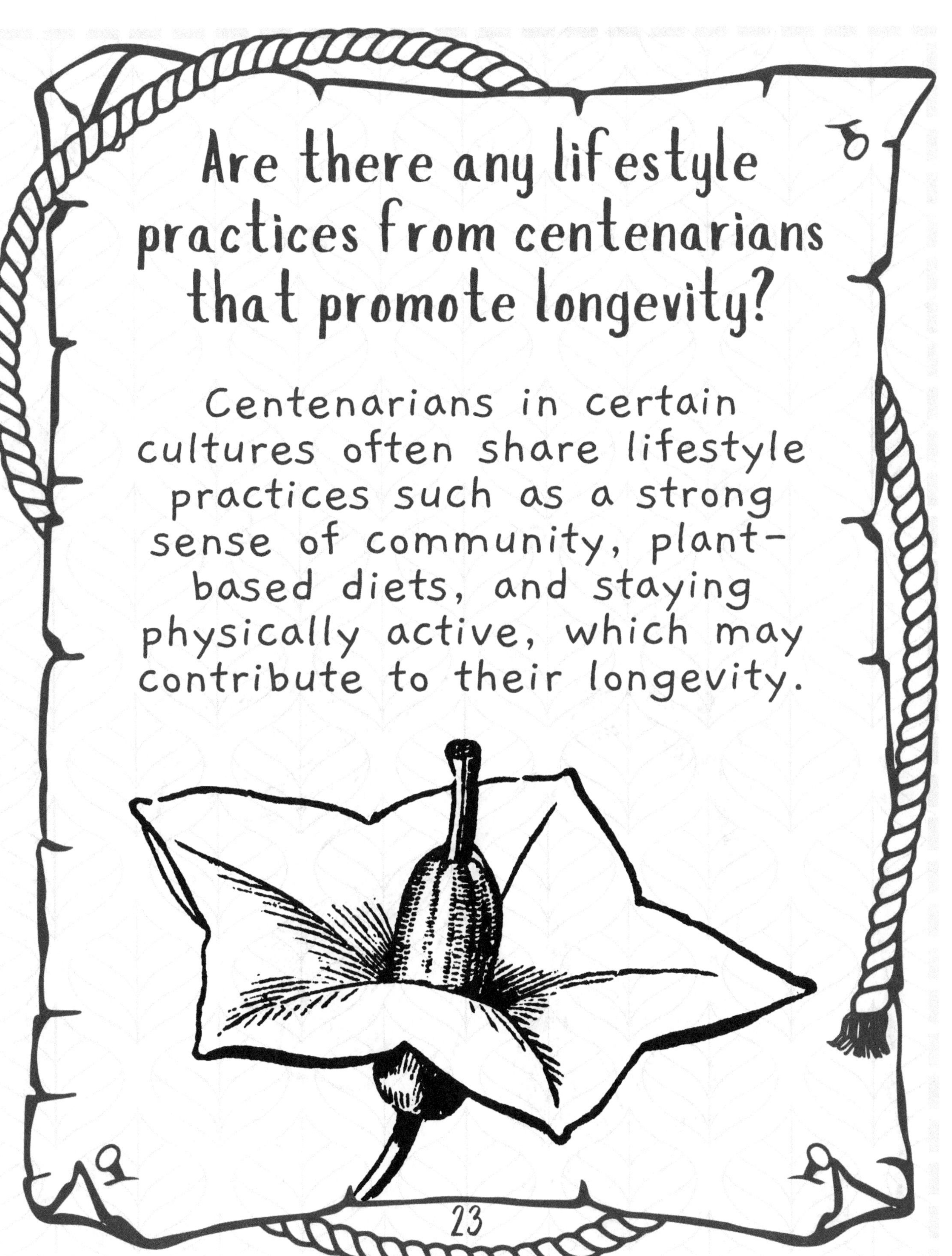

Can meditation and mindfulness practices affect longevity?

Meditation and mindfulness practices have been associated with stress reduction and improved mental well-being, potentially contributing to increased longevity.

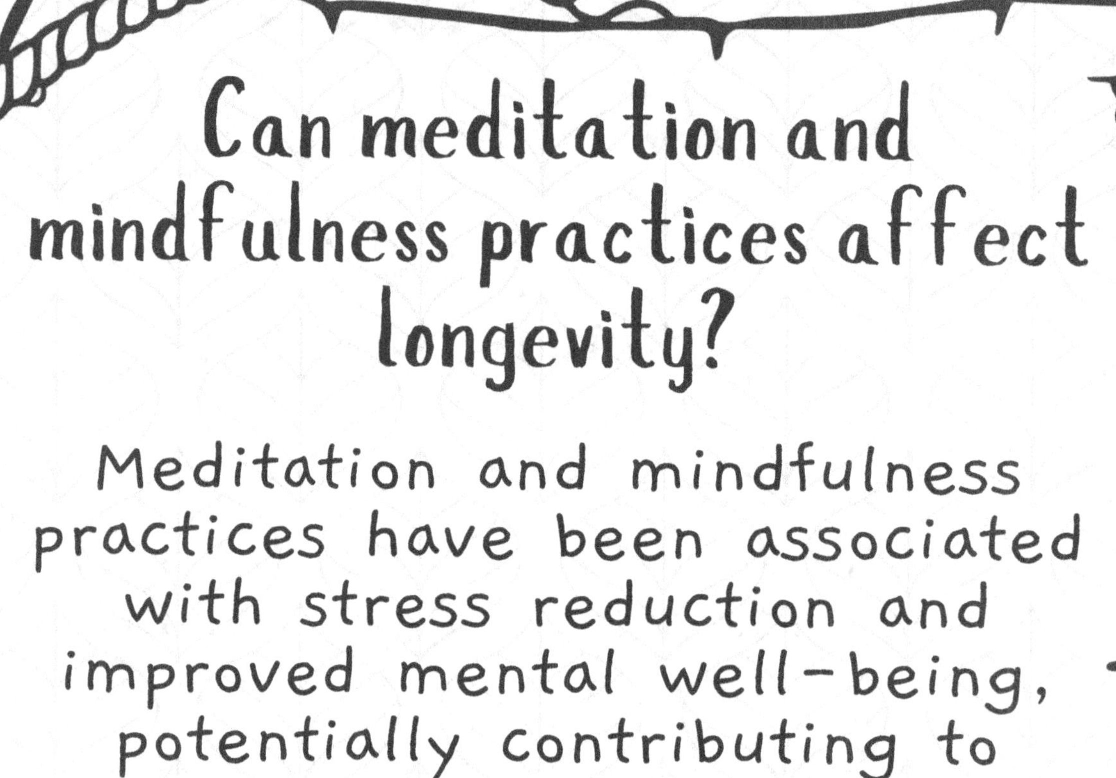

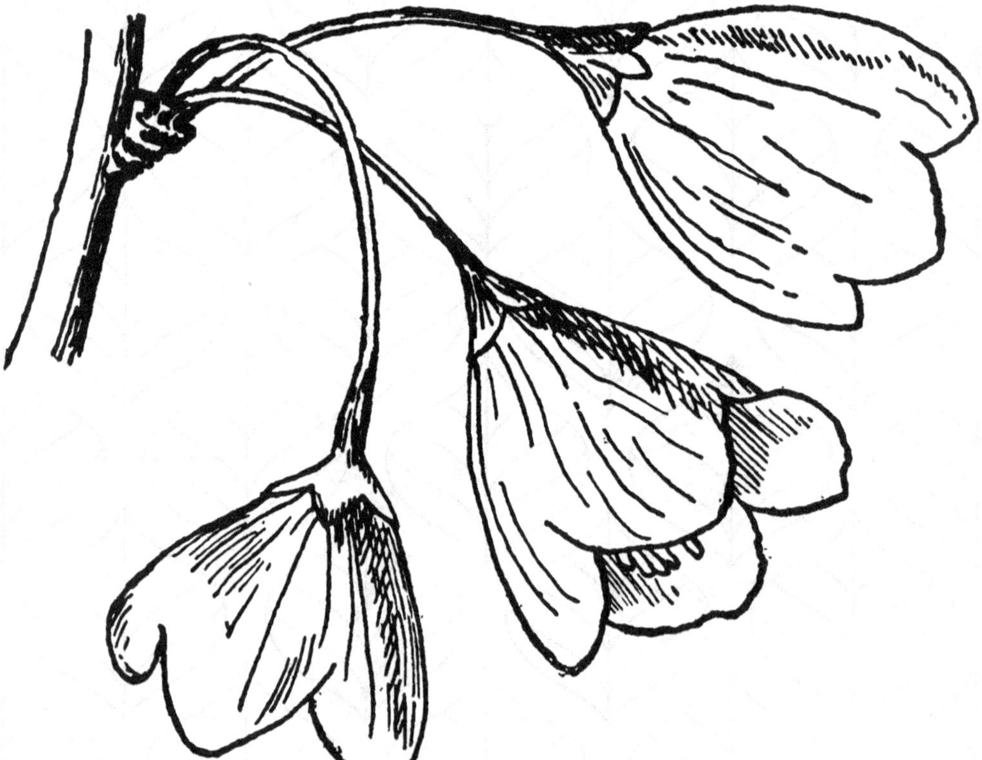

How does the immune system impact the aging process and longevity?

The immune system plays a crucial role in defending against diseases. As it ages, immune function can decline, influencing overall health and longevity.

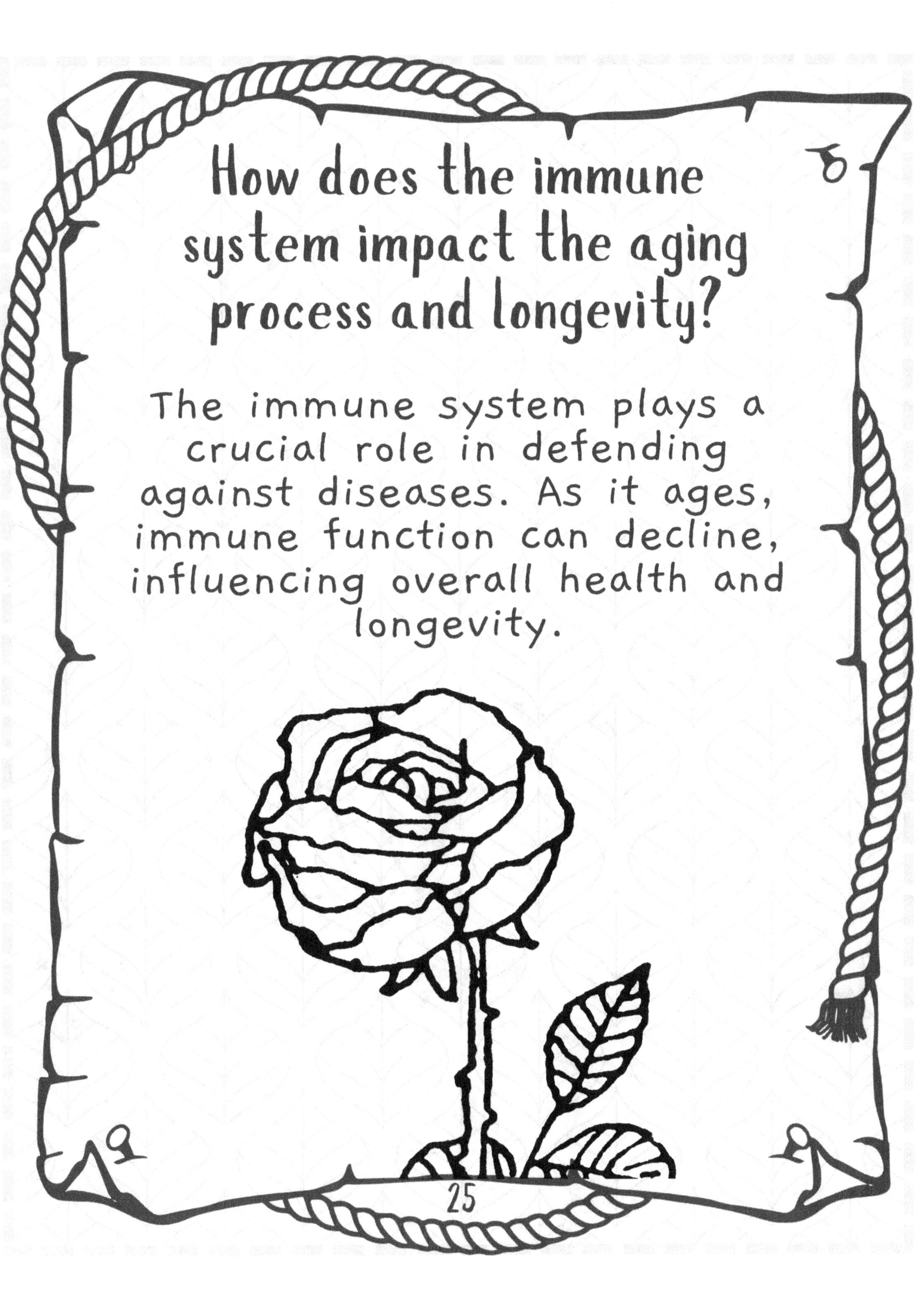

25

Are there any ethical considerations in the pursuit of longevity research?

Longevity research raises ethical questions related to genetic interventions, access to treatments, and the potential impact on societal structures.

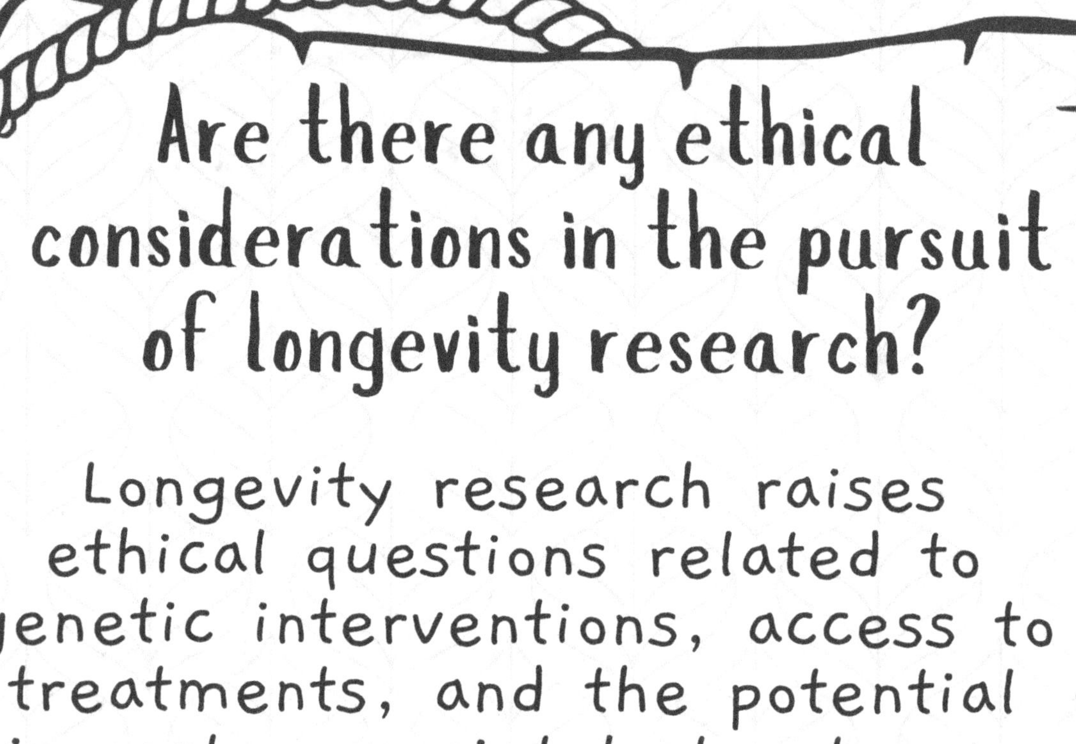

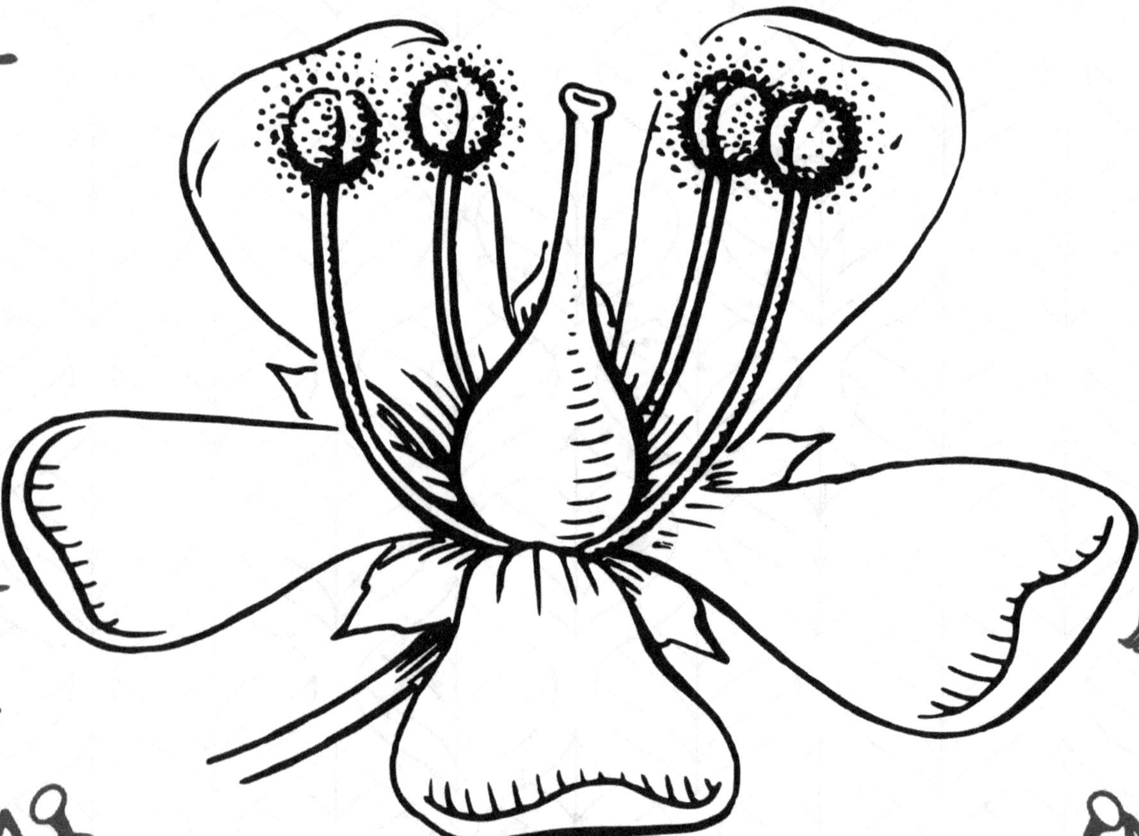

Can social and economic factors affect longevity disparities?

Socioeconomic factors, such as income, education, and access to healthcare, can contribute to disparities in longevity among different population groups.

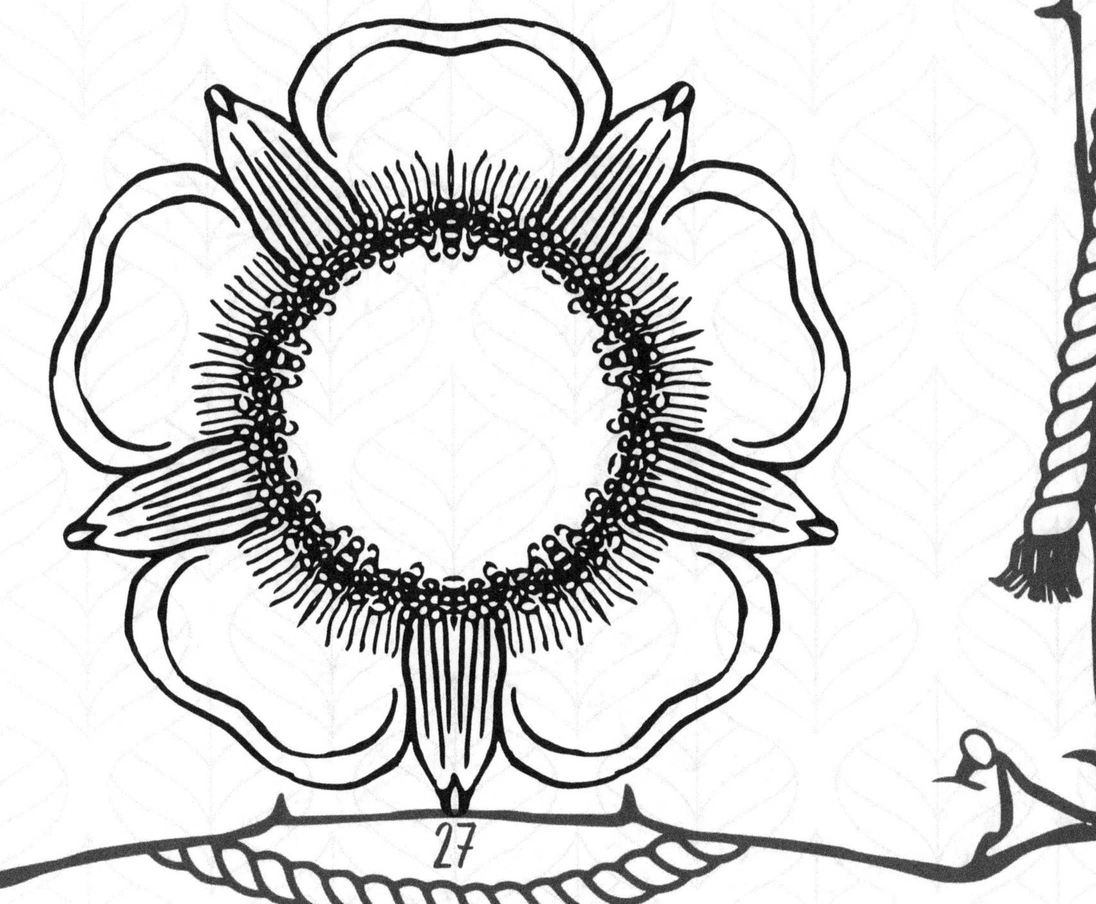

What role do hormones play in the aging process and longevity?

Hormones, including growth hormone and sex hormones, can influence the aging process, and hormone replacement therapy is an area of research in relation to longevity.

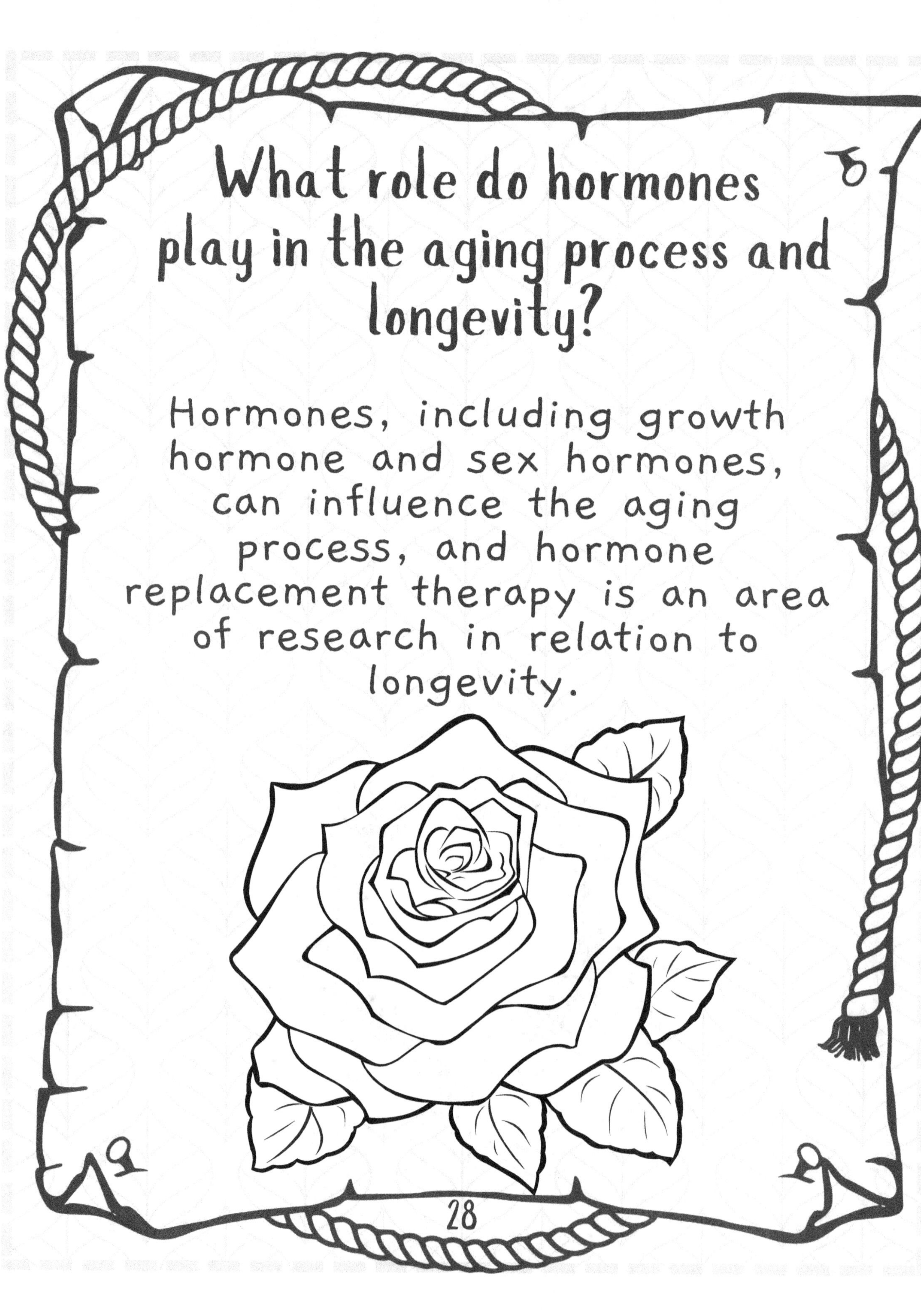

How does the concept of "healthspan" relate to longevity?

Healthspan refers to the period of life in which an individual remains healthy and free from serious diseases. Extending healthspan is a key focus in longevity research.

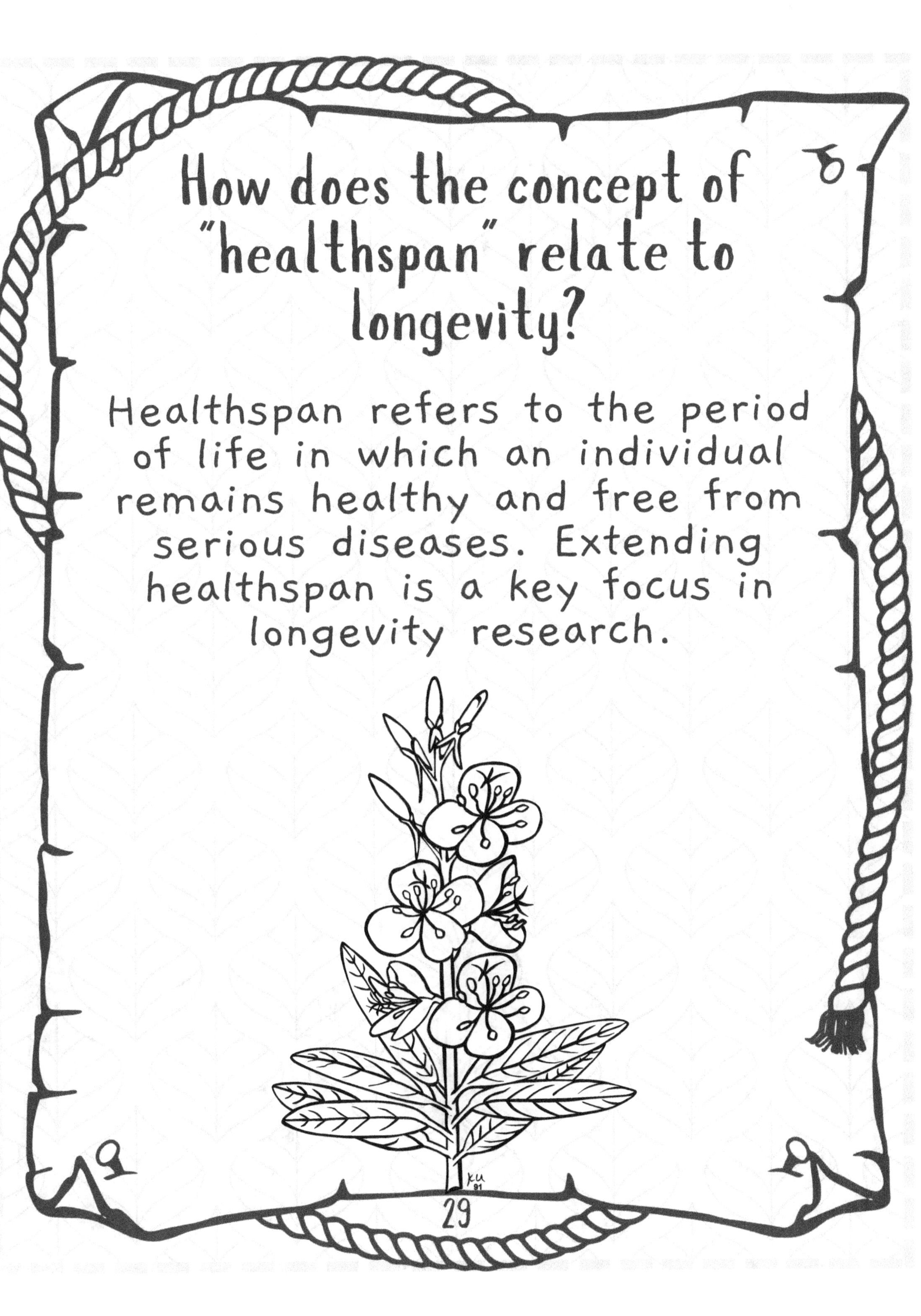

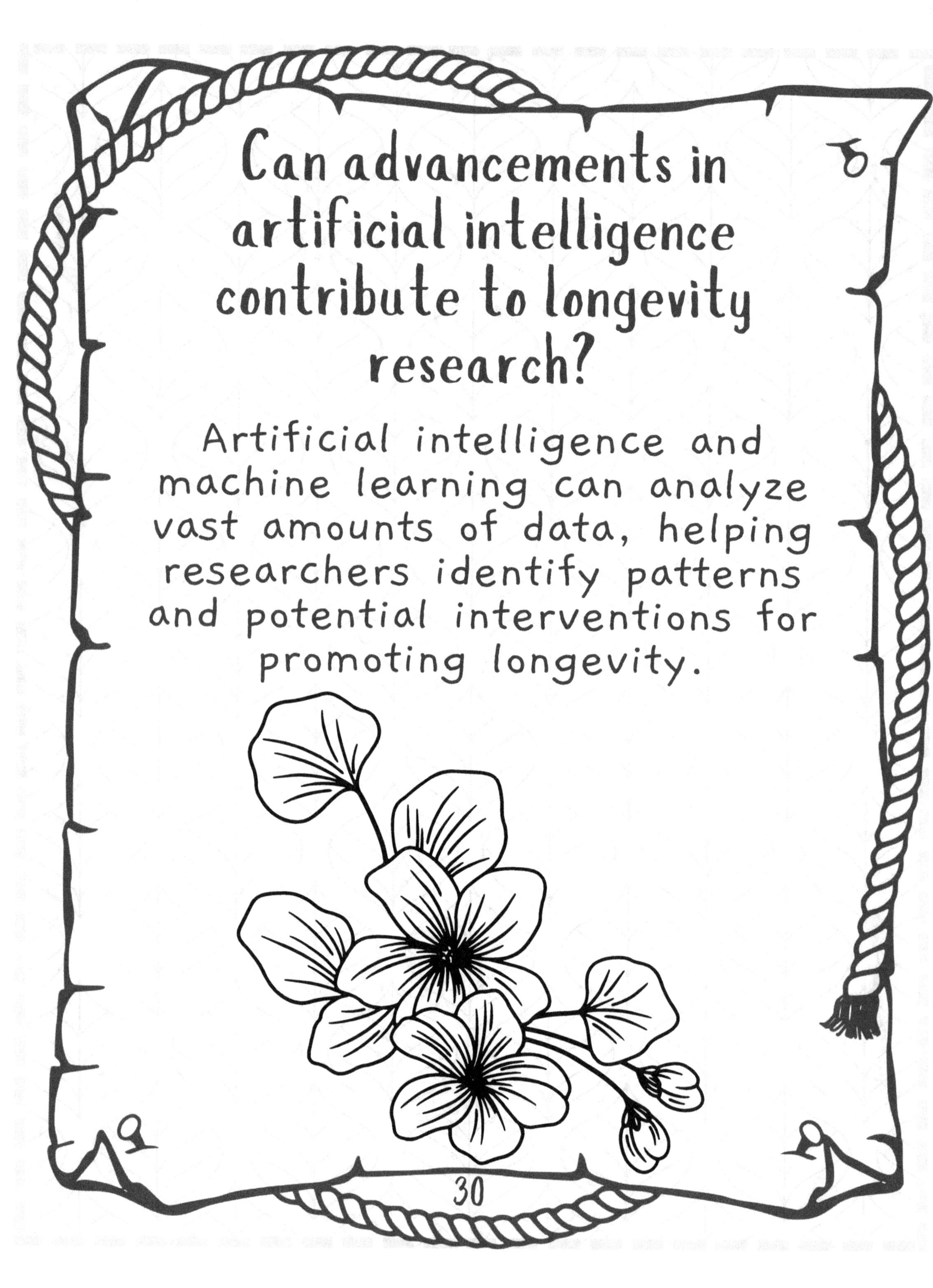

Can advancements in artificial intelligence contribute to longevity research?

Artificial intelligence and machine learning can analyze vast amounts of data, helping researchers identify patterns and potential interventions for promoting longevity.

How does chronic inflammation impact aging and longevity?

Chronic inflammation is linked to various age-related diseases. Managing inflammation through lifestyle and medical interventions may positively influence longevity.

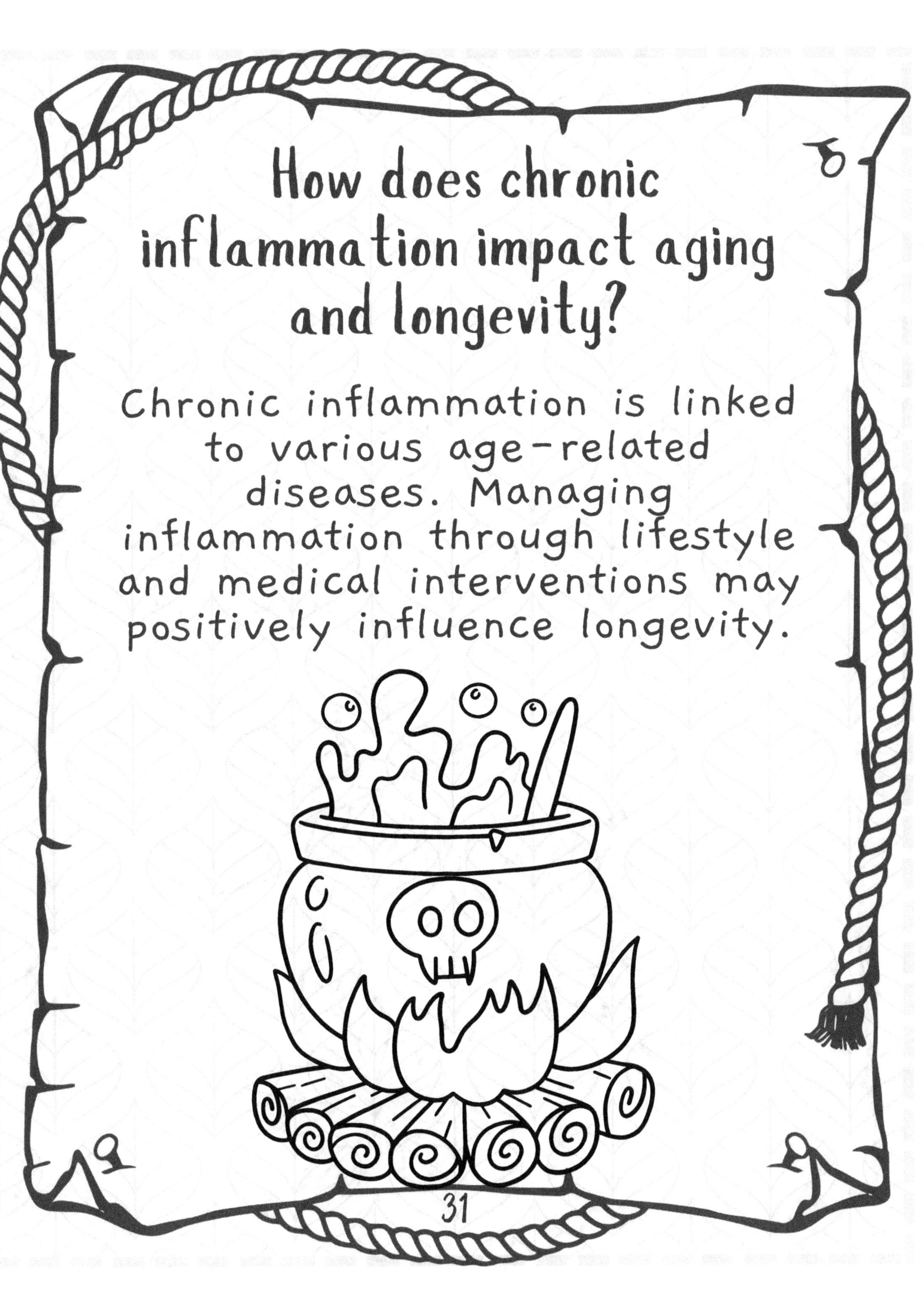

Are there any cultural variations in attitudes toward aging and longevity?

Cultural attitudes toward aging vary, impacting lifestyle choices, healthcare practices, and societal support systems, all of which can influence longevity.

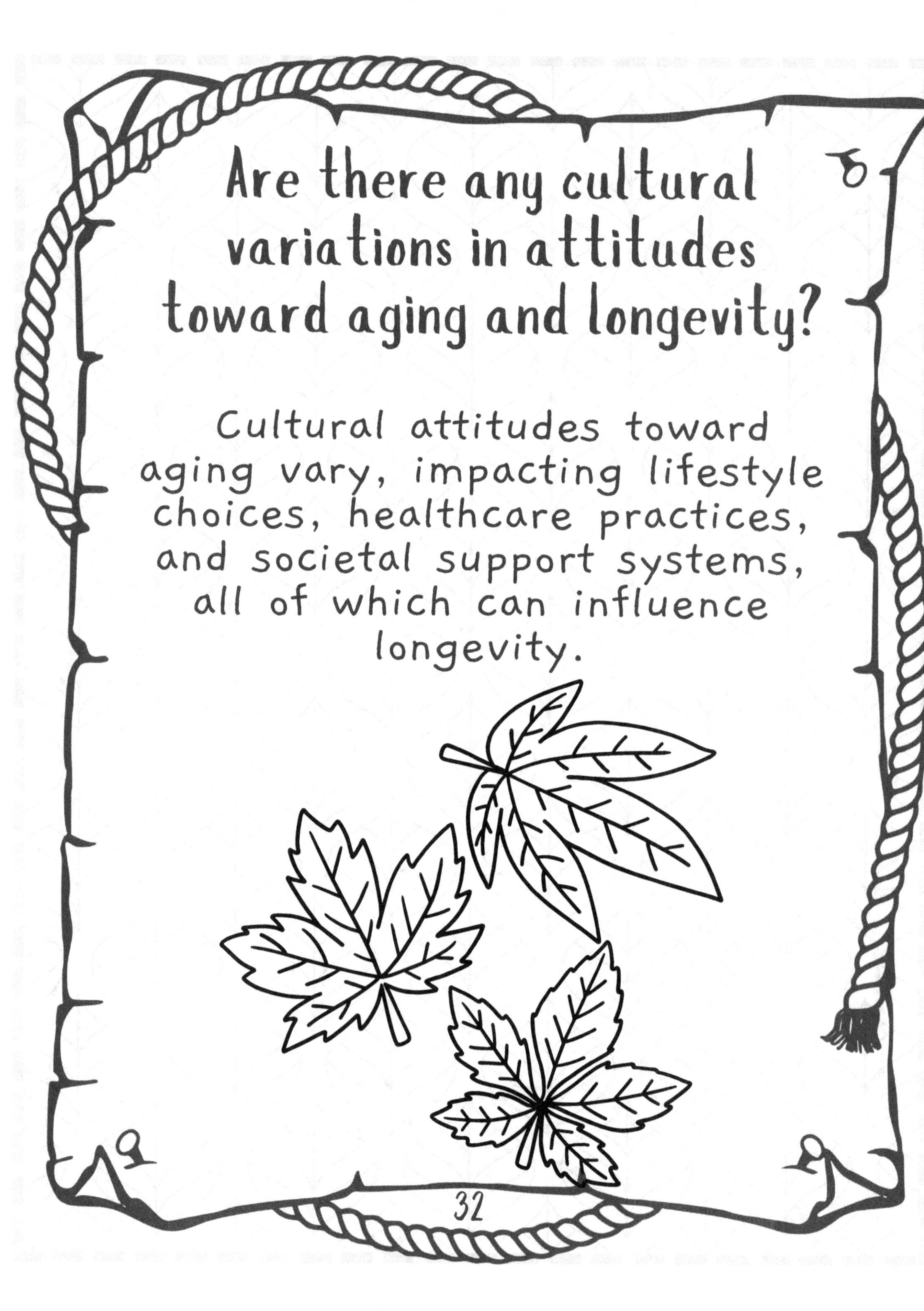

Can advancements in nanotechnology play a role in longevity research?

Nanotechnology has the potential to revolutionize medicine, including targeted drug delivery and diagnostics, contributing to advancements in longevity research.

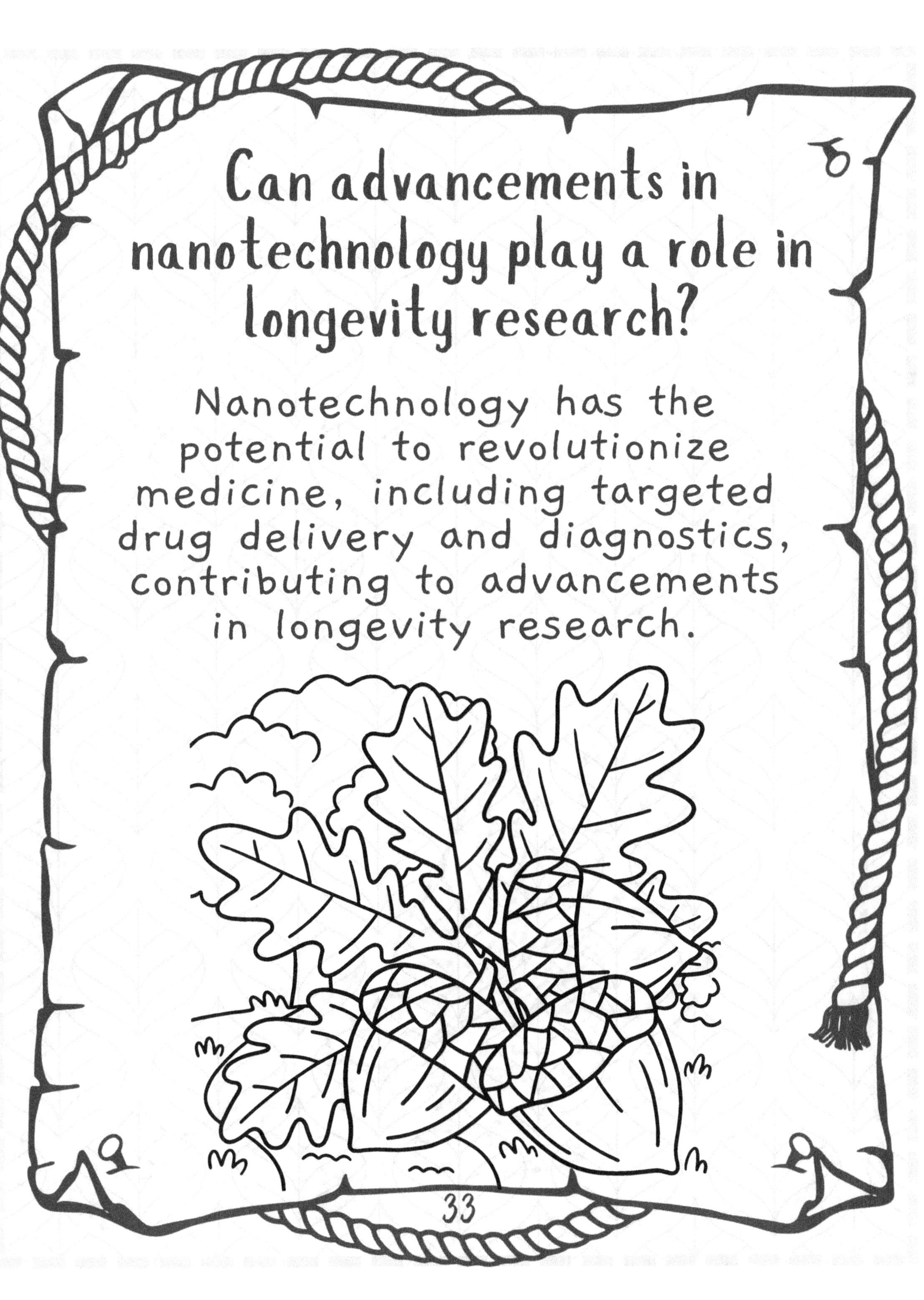

How does the concept of "resilience" relate to longevity?

Resilience, the ability to adapt and bounce back from challenges, is associated with better health outcomes and may contribute to increased longevity.

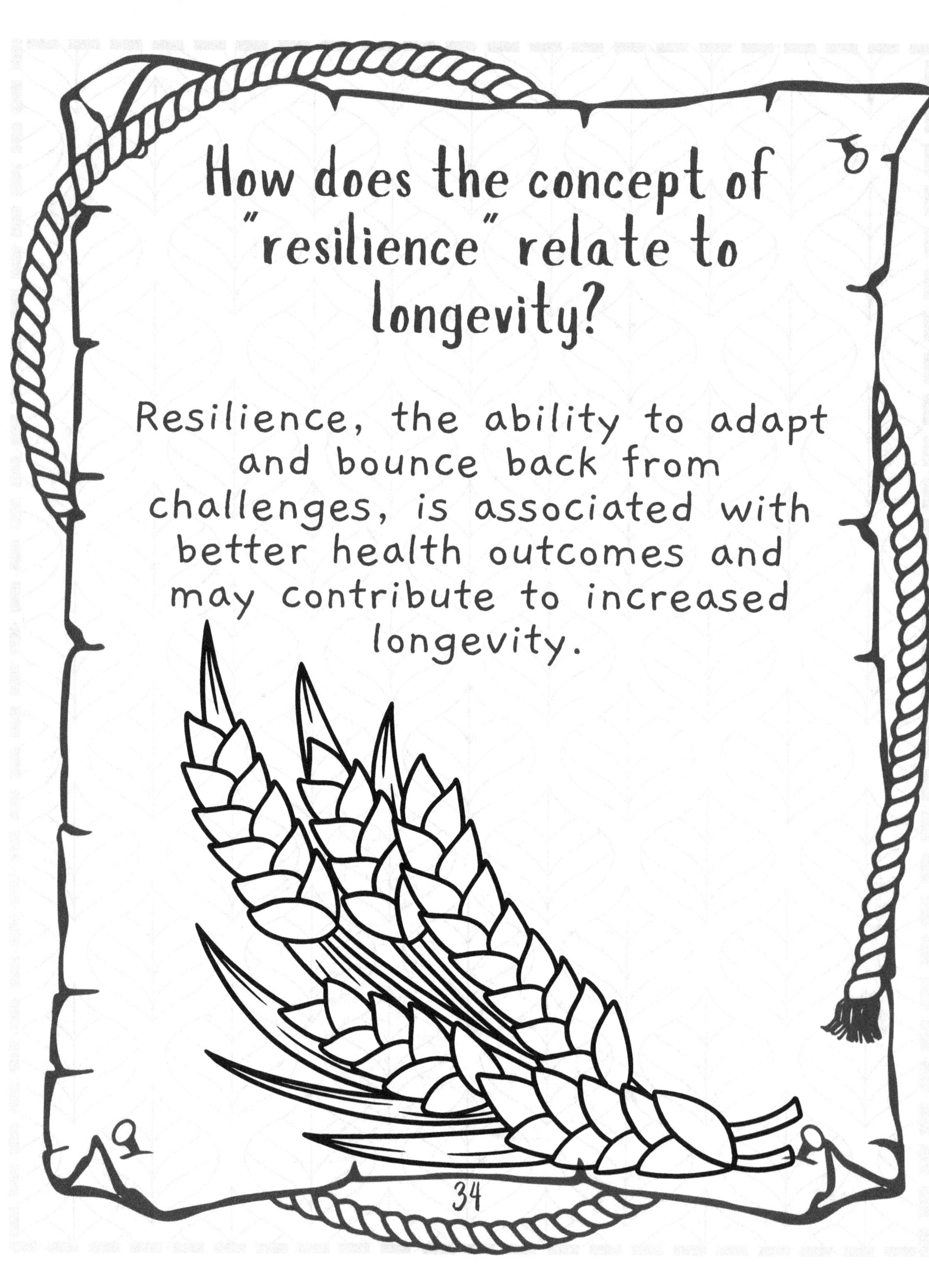

Can studying the aging process in other species provide insights into human longevity?

Research on model organisms like mice and certain non-human primates helps scientists understand fundamental biological processes related to aging, offering insights into human longevity.

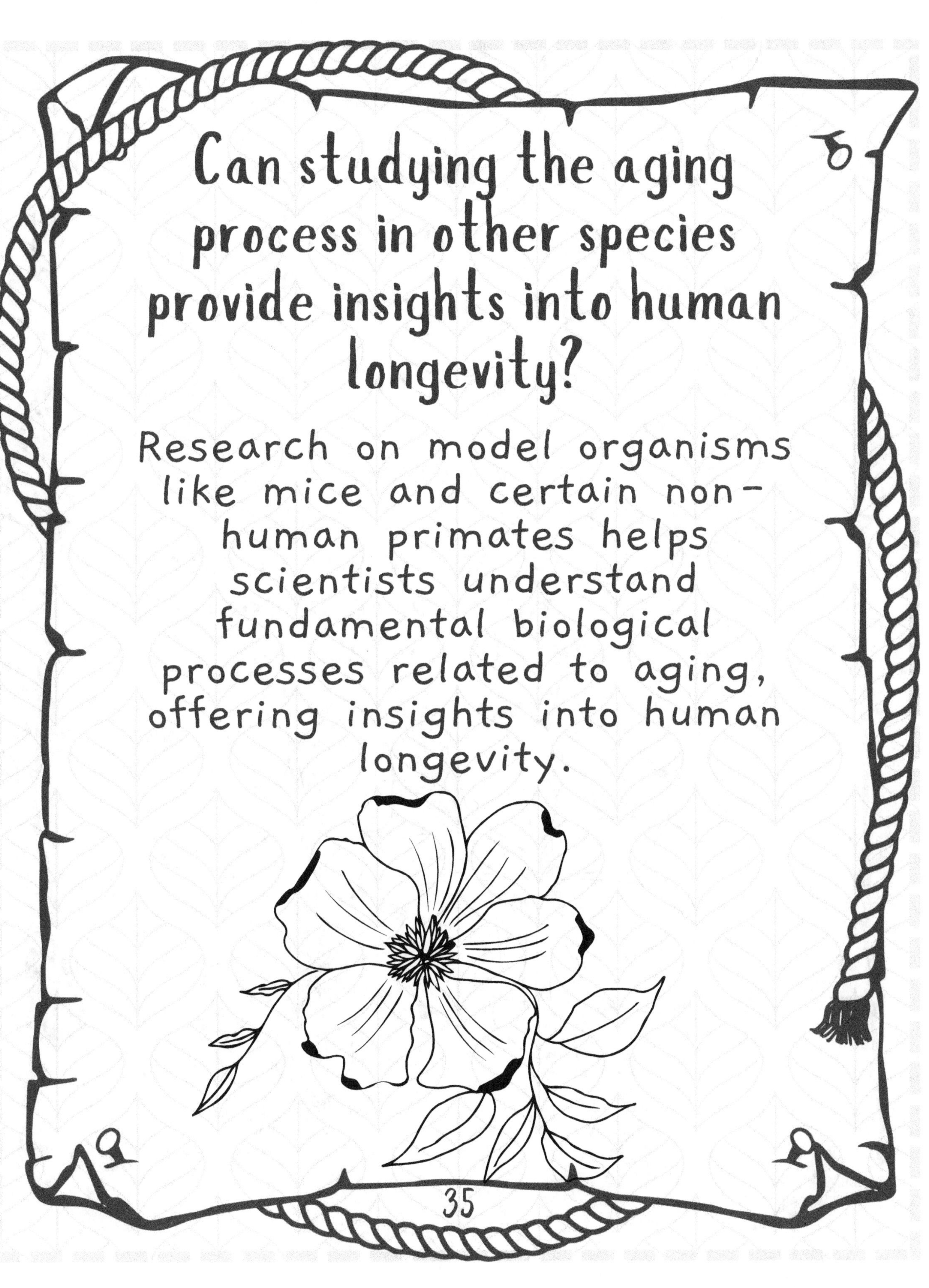

How does the concept of "senescence" relate to aging and longevity?

Cellular senescence refers to the state in which cells cease to divide. Accumulation of senescent cells is associated with aging and age-related diseases, making it a focus in longevity research.

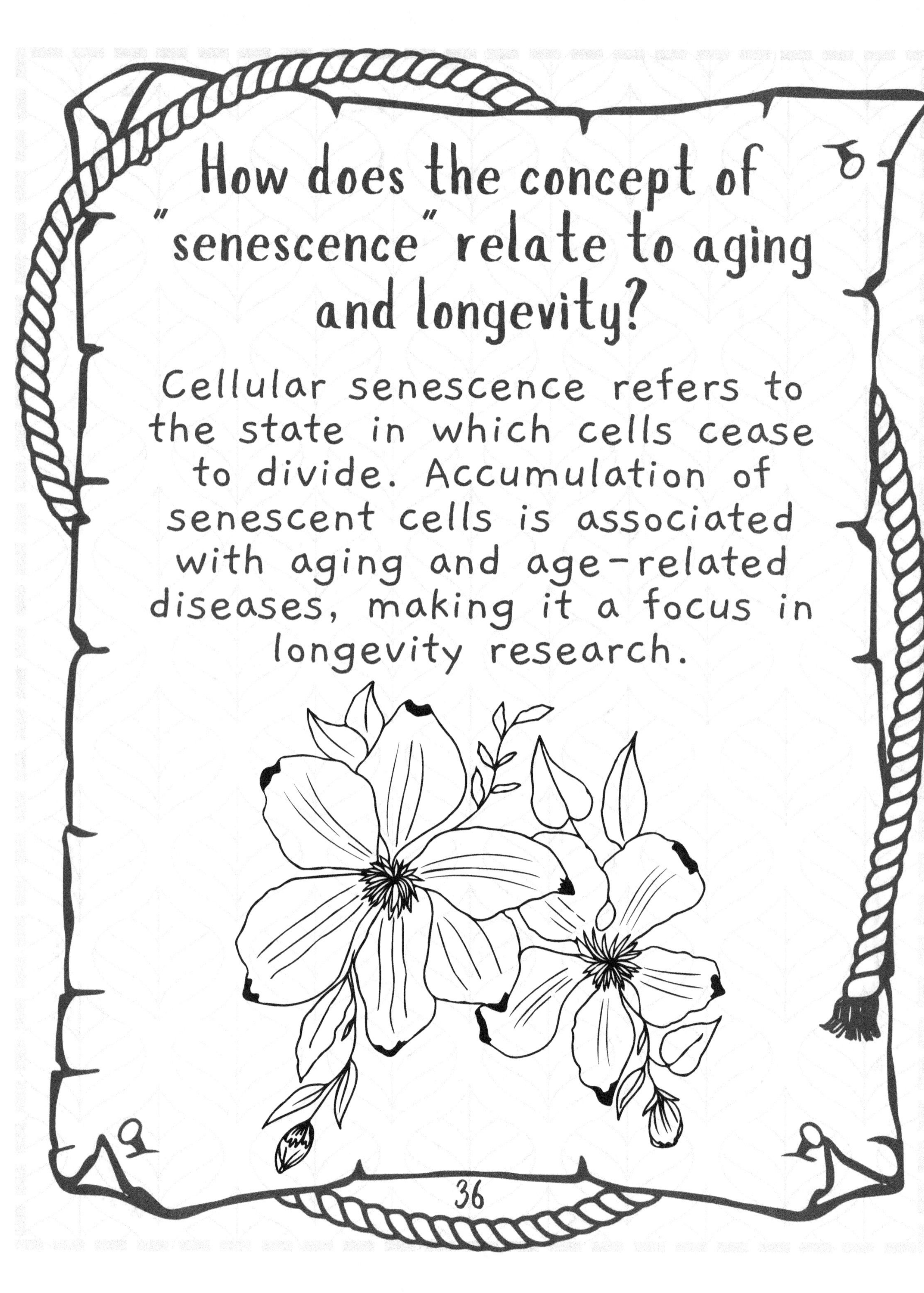

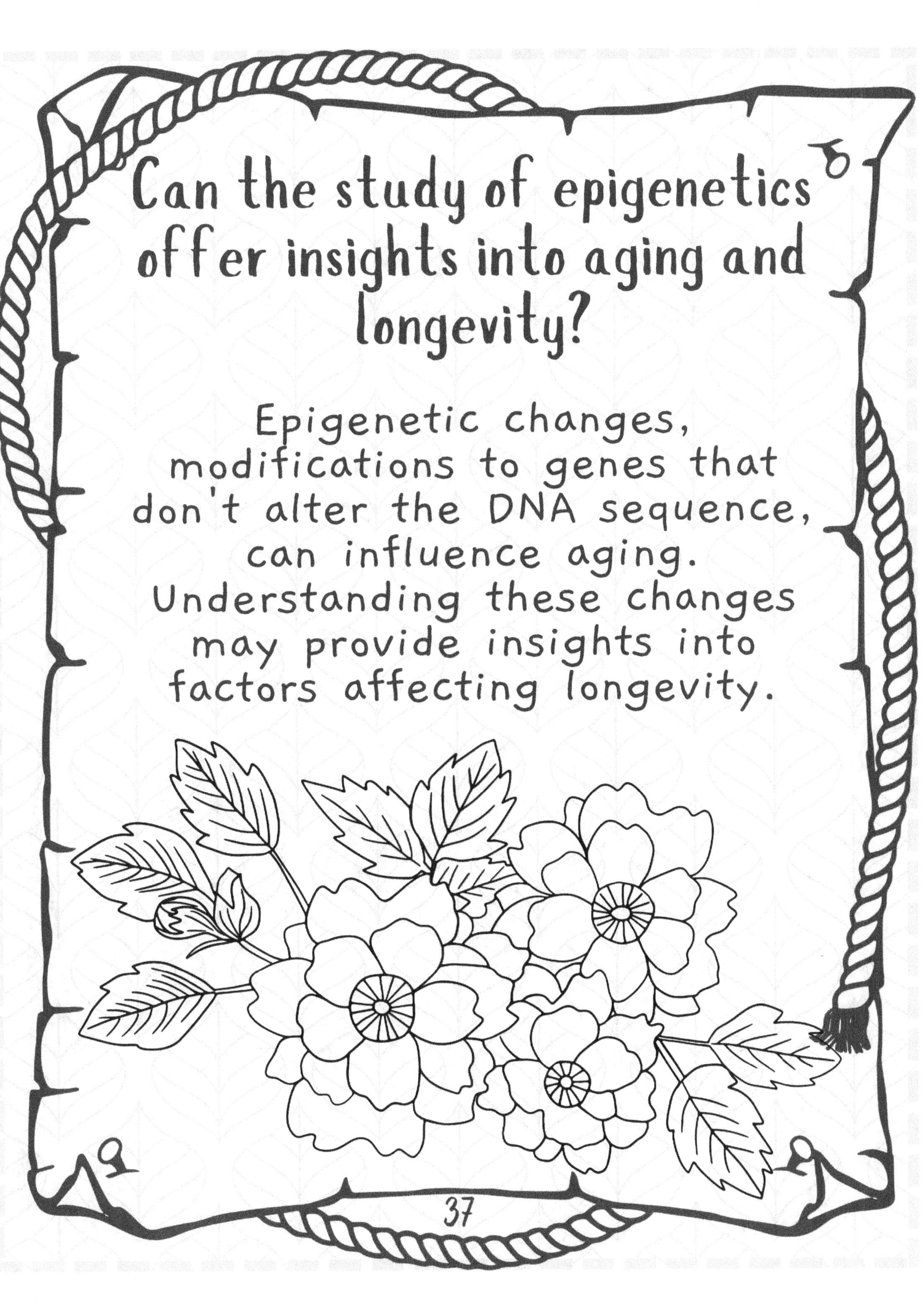

Can the study of epigenetics offer insights into aging and longevity?

Epigenetic changes, modifications to genes that don't alter the DNA sequence, can influence aging. Understanding these changes may provide insights into factors affecting longevity.

How does environmental sustainability connect with longevity considerations?

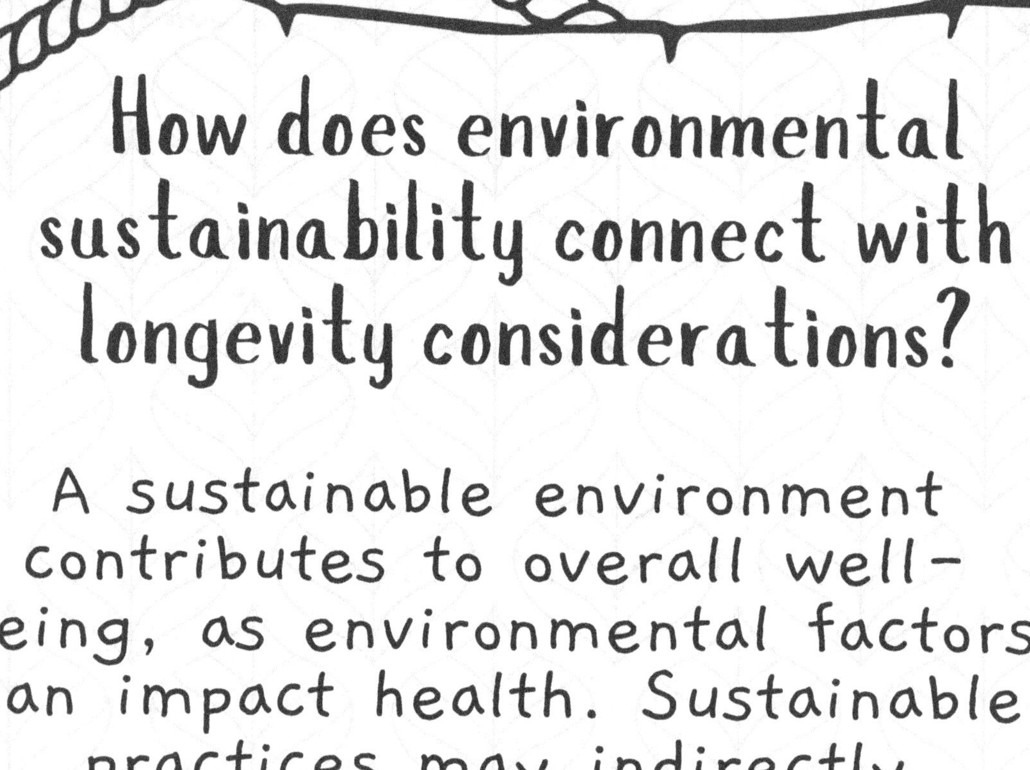

A sustainable environment contributes to overall well-being, as environmental factors can impact health. Sustainable practices may indirectly support longevity.

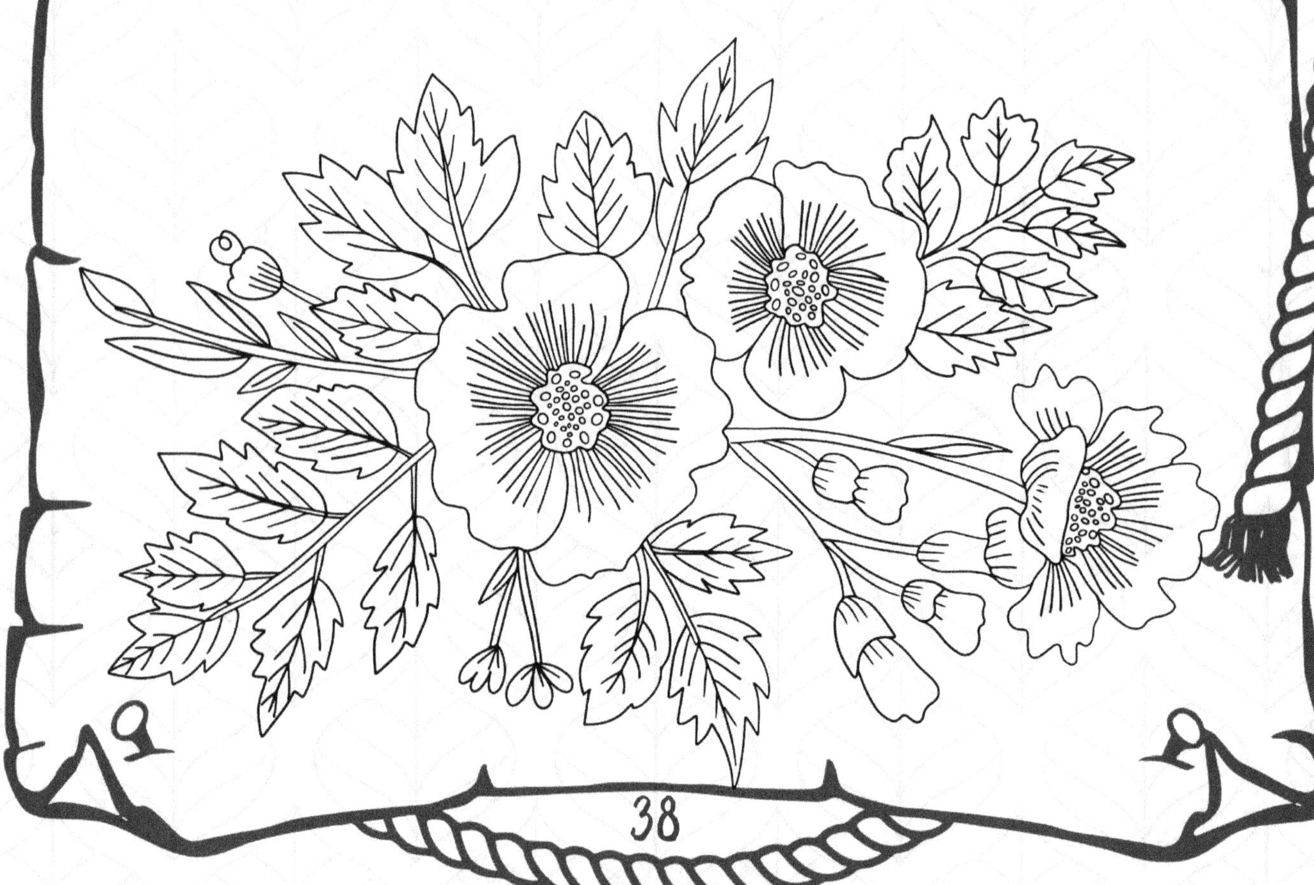

Is there a connection between educational attainment and longevity?

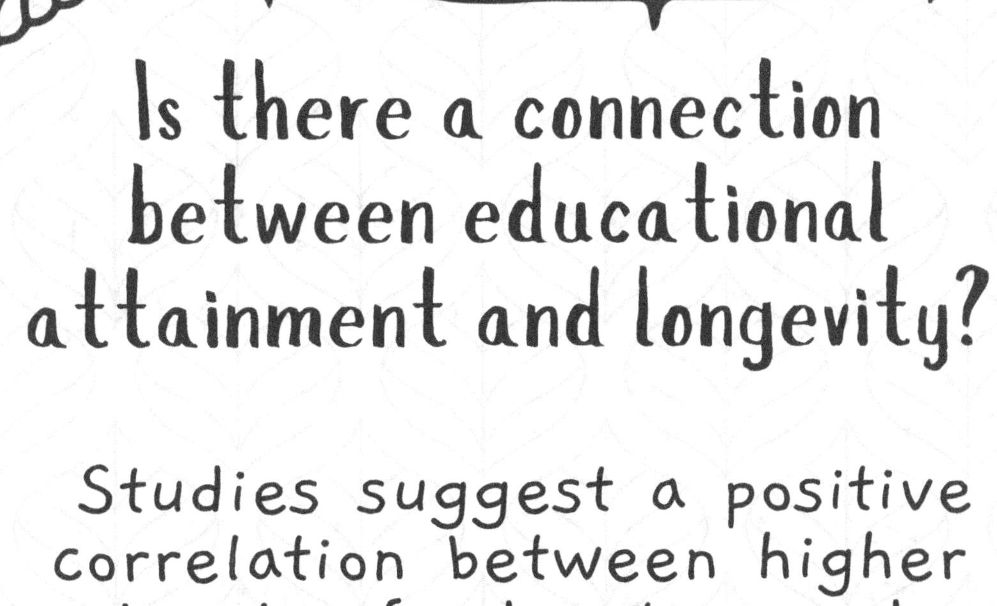

Studies suggest a positive correlation between higher levels of education and increased longevity, possibly due to better health knowledge and access to resources.

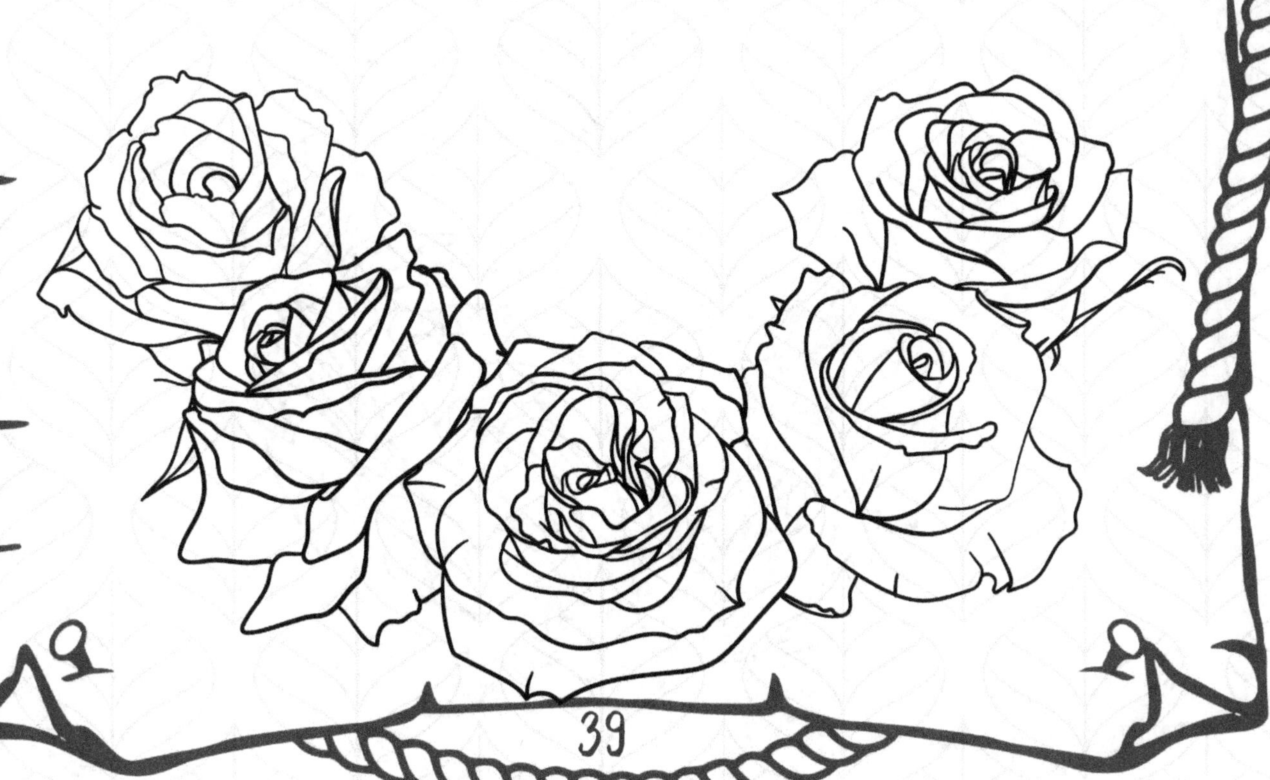

Can stem cell research play a role in extending lifespan or treating age-related diseases?

Stem cells have the potential to regenerate damaged tissues. Research in this field explores applications for treating age-related conditions and promoting longevity.

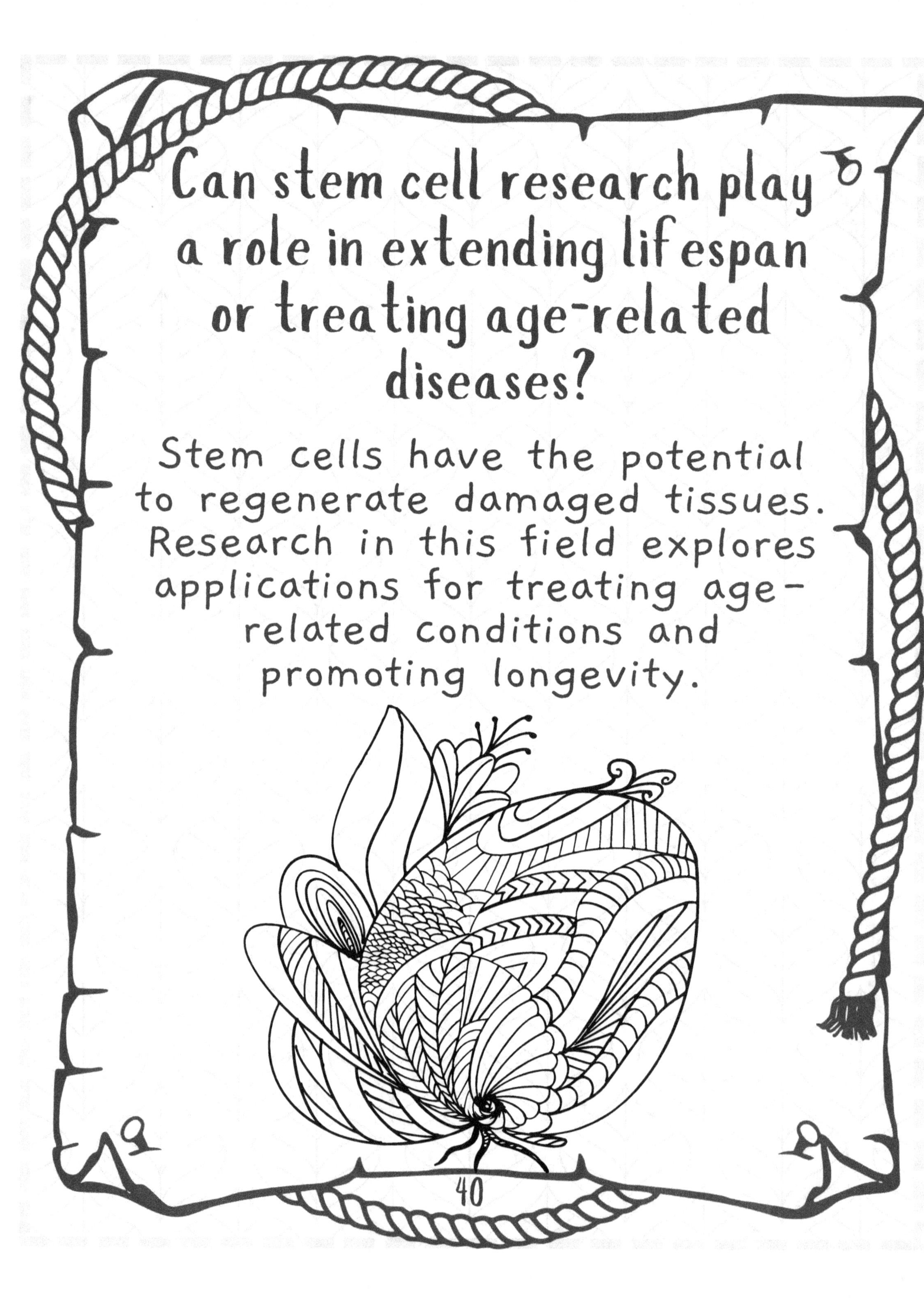

How do lifestyle interventions, such as intermittent fasting, impact longevity?

A: Some studies suggest that intermittent fasting and other dietary interventions may influence cellular repair processes and potentially extend lifespan. However, more research is needed.

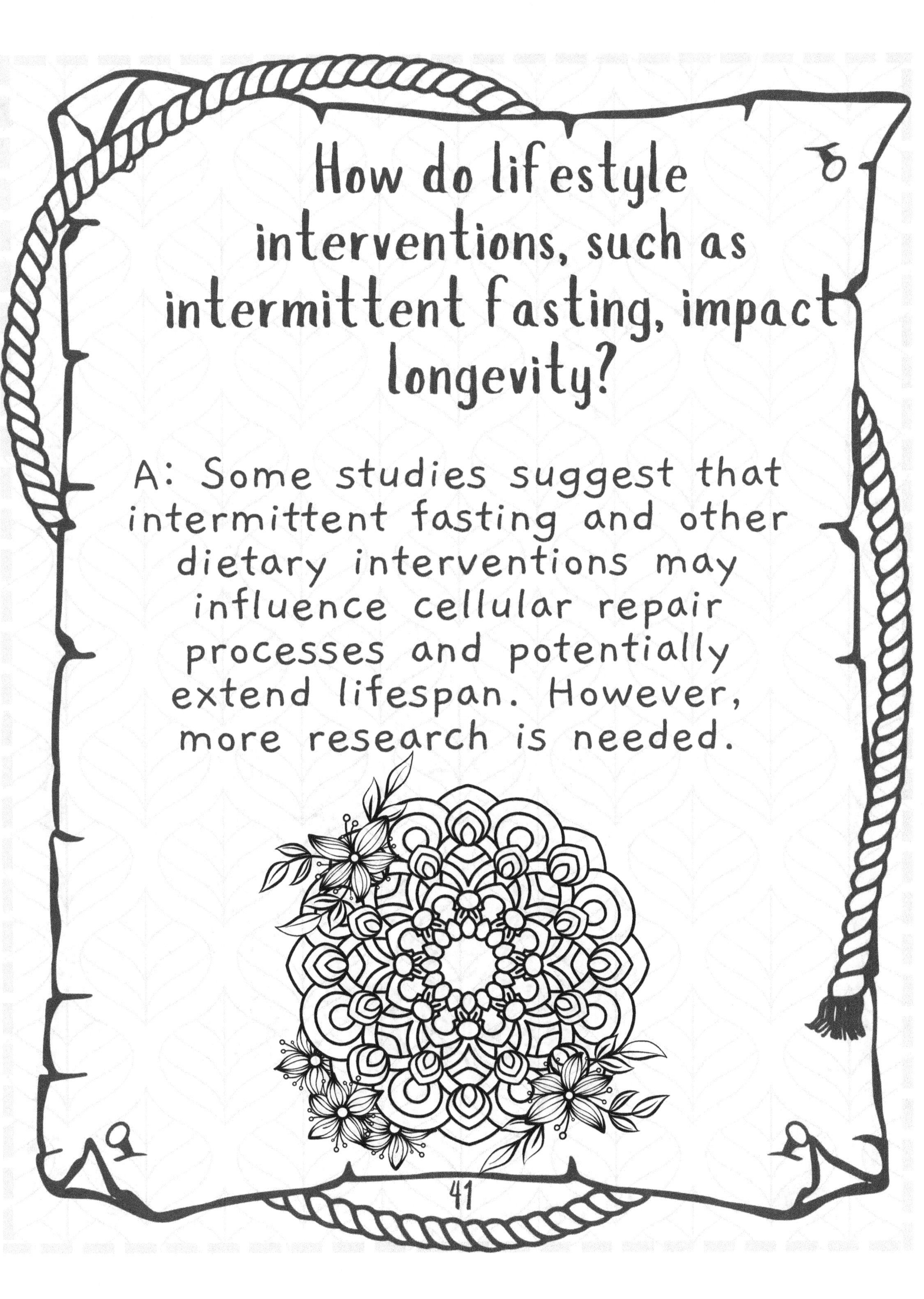

Can the microbiome of extremophiles offer insights into longevity mechanisms?

A: Studying extremophiles' microbiomes, organisms thriving in extreme conditions, may provide insights into biological adaptations that could be relevant to longevity research.

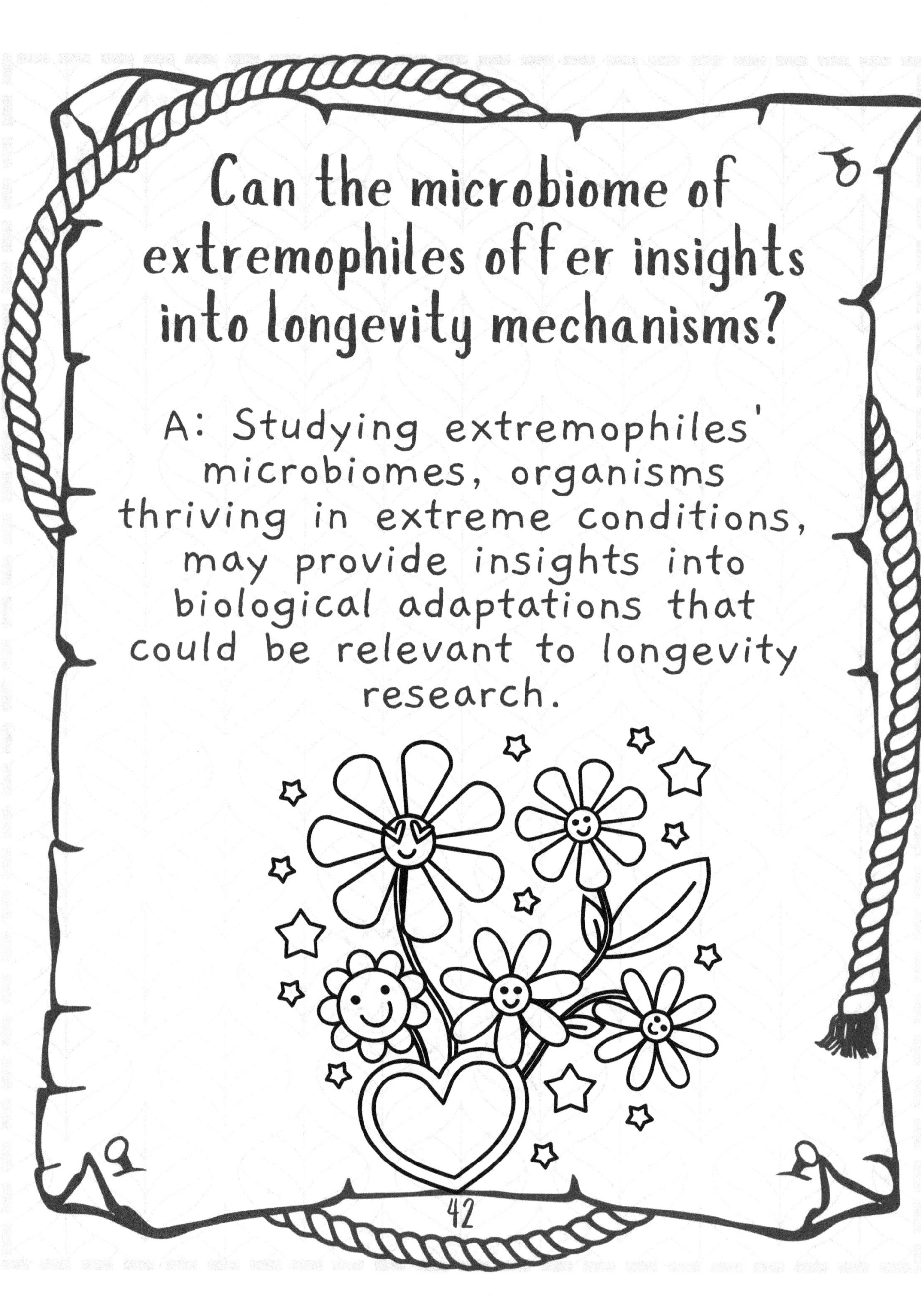

How does the circadian rhythm affect aging and longevity?

Disruptions to the circadian rhythm, the body's internal clock, are associated with aging. Maintaining a healthy circadian rhythm is considered important for longevity.

Can advancements in cryonics impact perceptions of life extension and longevity?

Cryonics involves preserving bodies at low temperatures with the hope of future revival. While speculative, it raises ethical and philosophical questions about life extension.

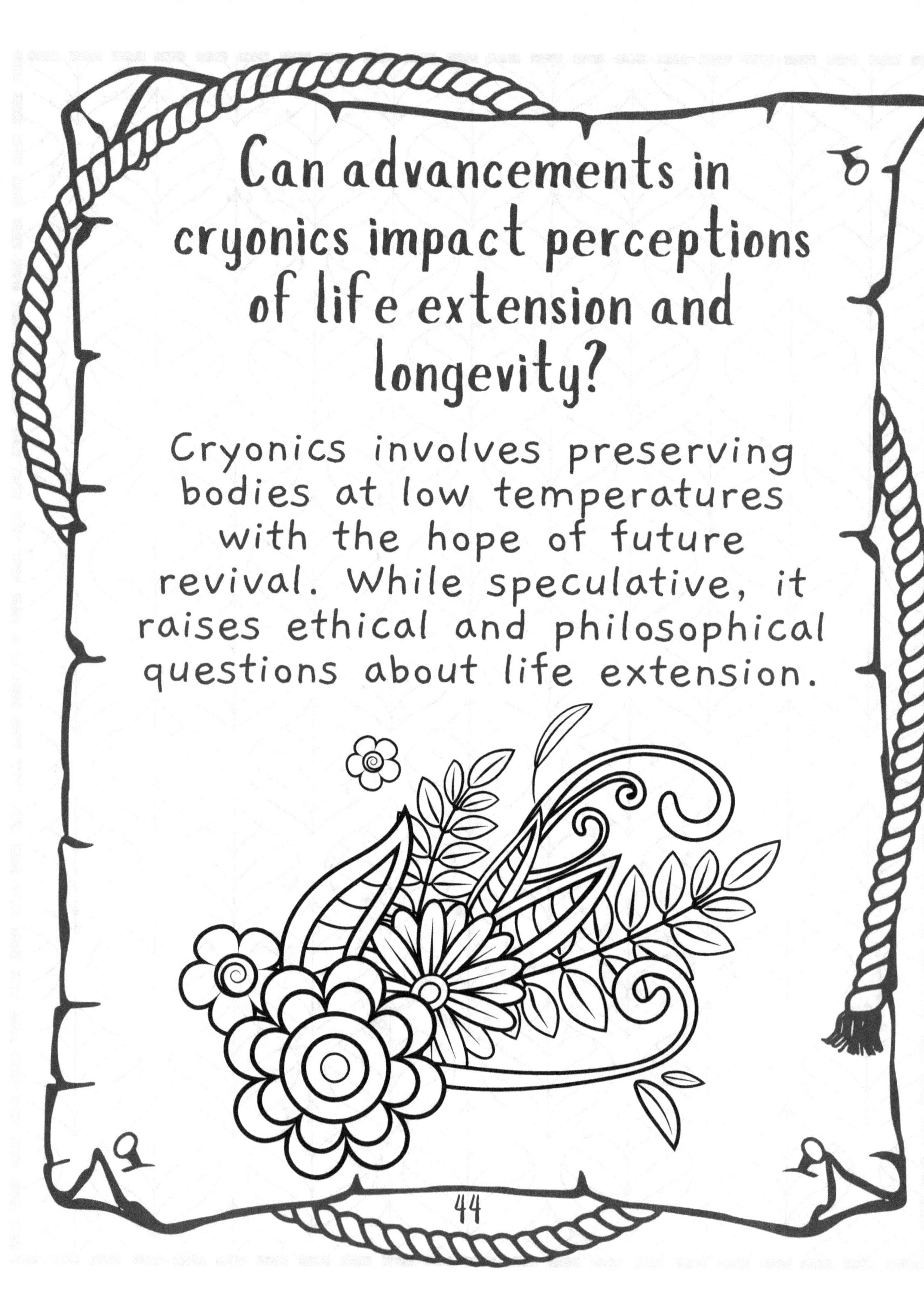

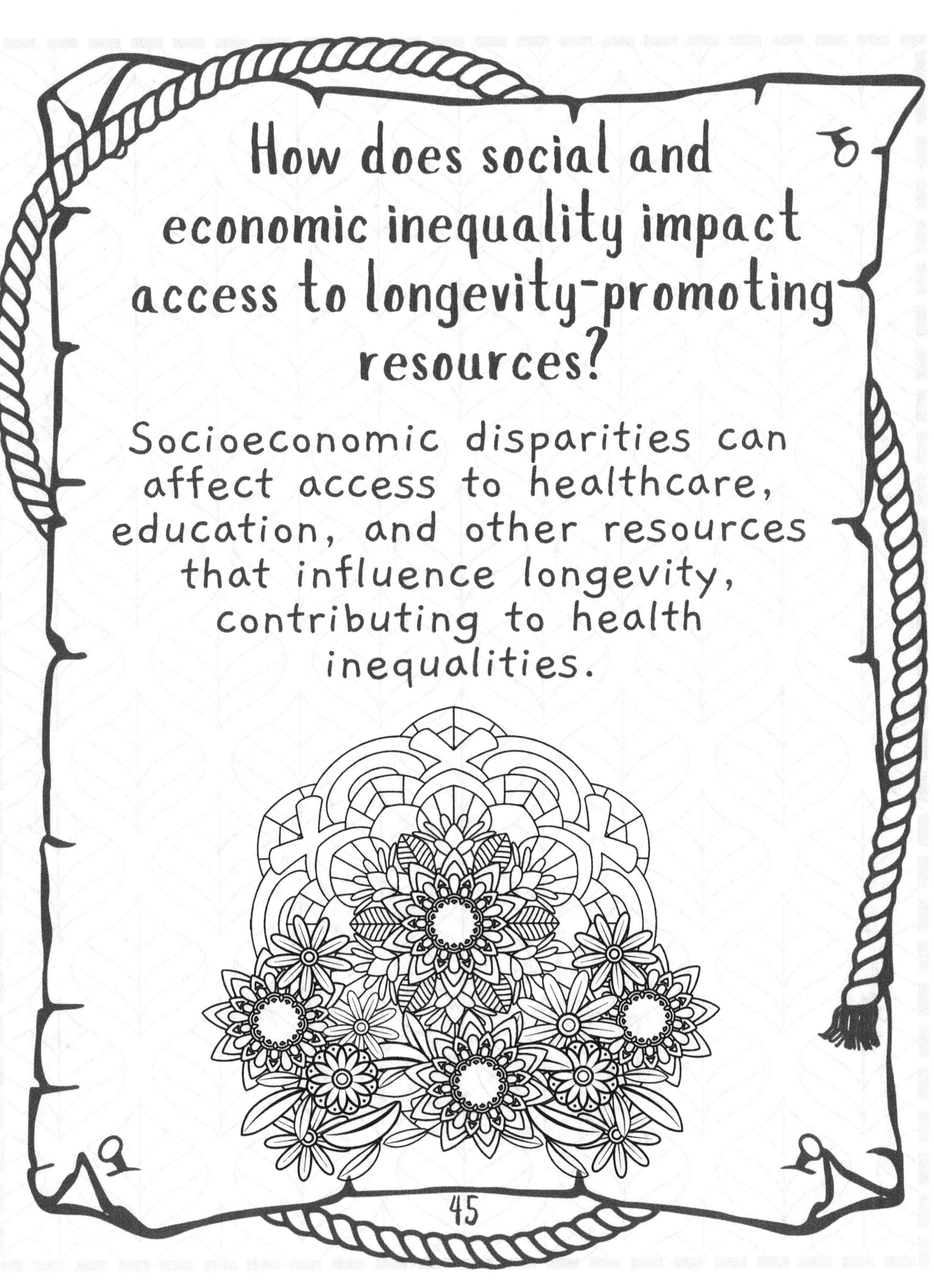

How does social and economic inequality impact access to longevity-promoting resources?

Socioeconomic disparities can affect access to healthcare, education, and other resources that influence longevity, contributing to health inequalities.

Can artificial intelligence predict an individual's risk of age-related diseases and impact longevity?

AI models analyzing health data can predict disease risks and suggest personalized interventions, potentially impacting longevity by enabling proactive healthcare.

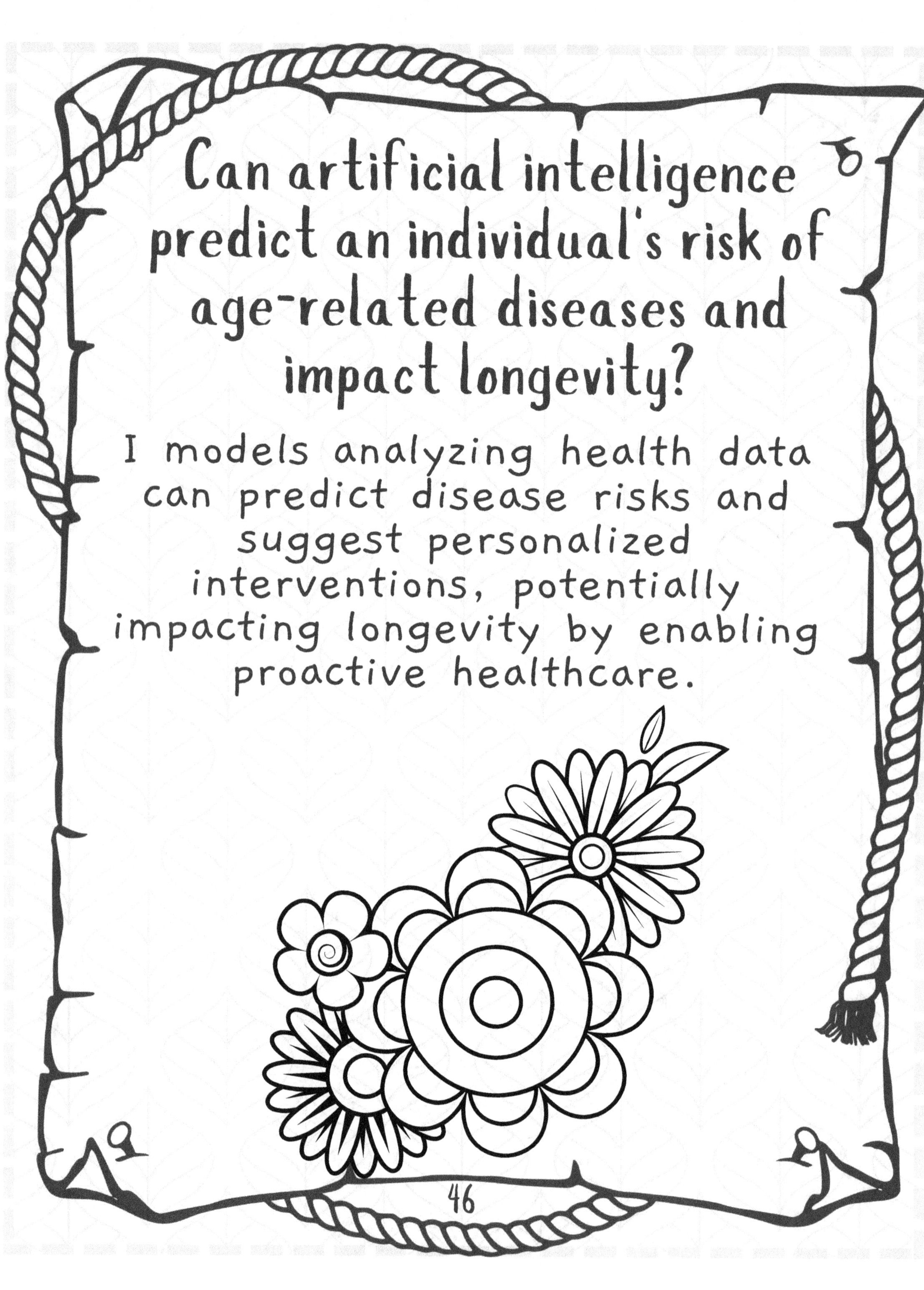

How does the availability of clean water and sanitation impact global longevity rates?

Access to clean water and sanitation is crucial for preventing diseases. Improved public health infrastructure contributes to increased longevity globally.

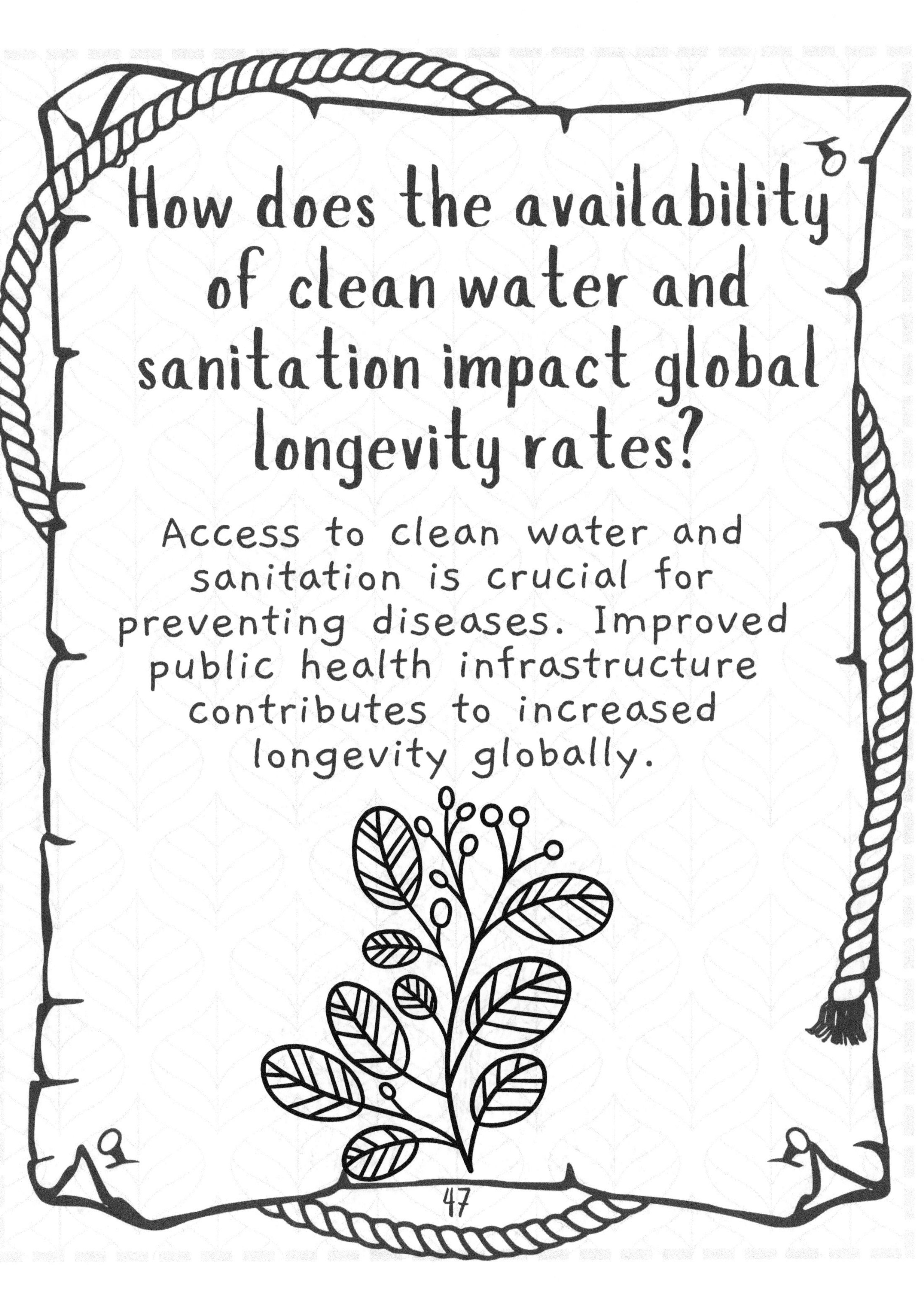

What role do vaccinations play in promoting longevity and preventing age-related diseases?

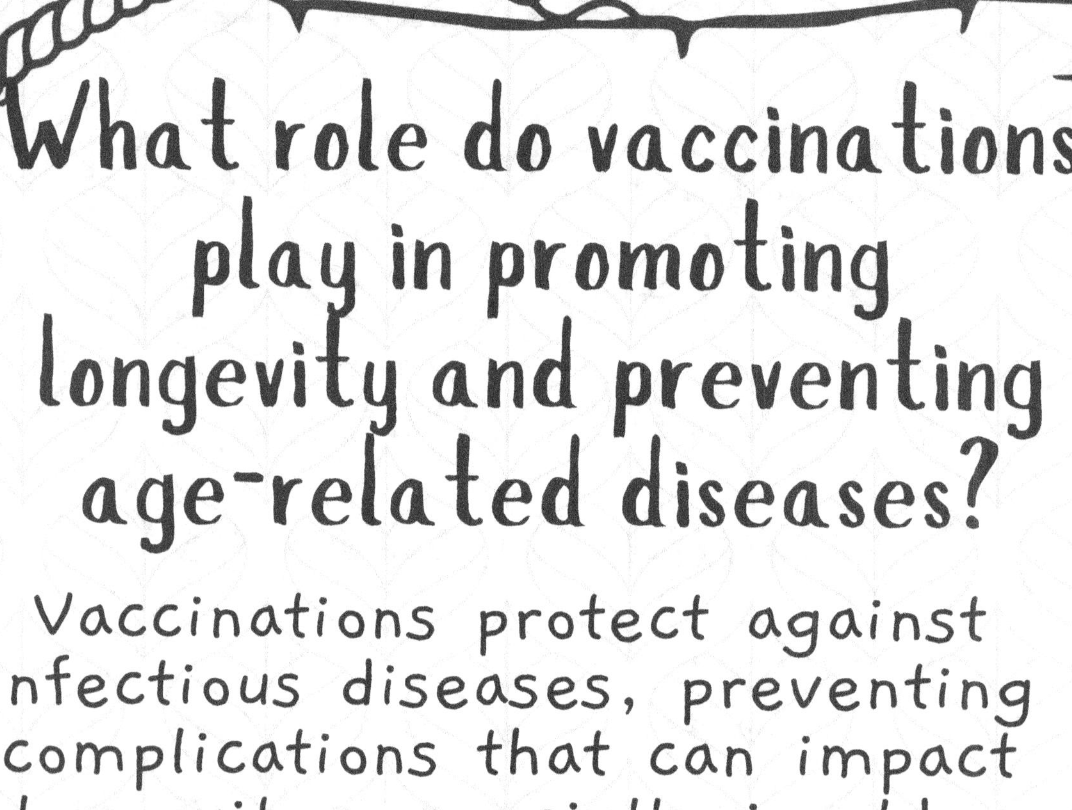

Vaccinations protect against infectious diseases, preventing complications that can impact longevity, especially in older adults with weakened immune systems.

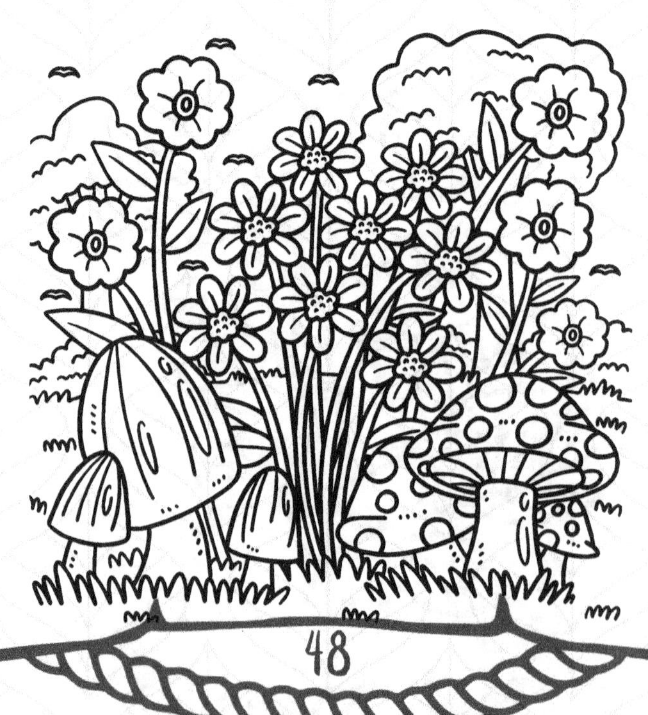

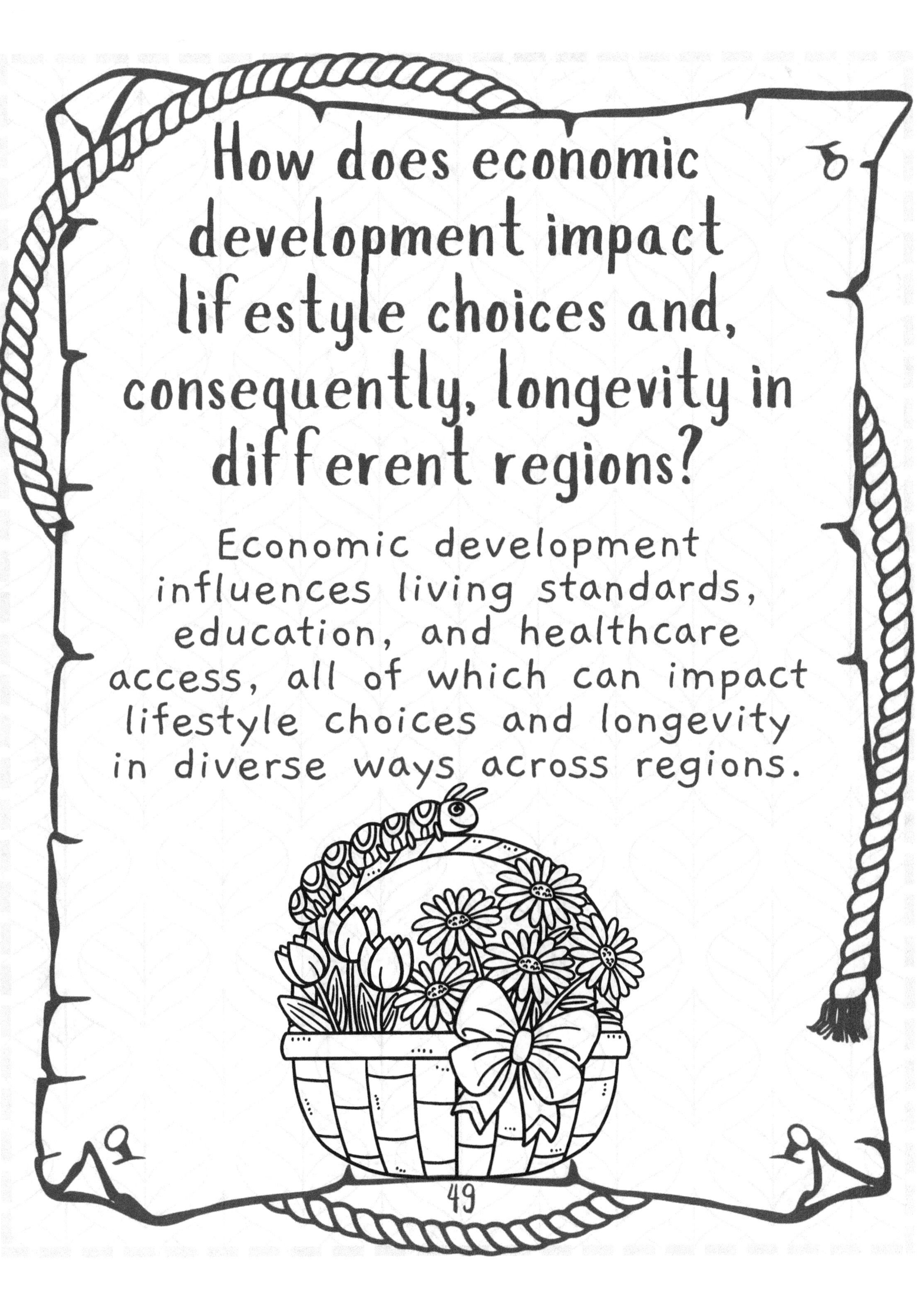

How does economic development impact lifestyle choices and, consequently, longevity in different regions?

Economic development influences living standards, education, and healthcare access, all of which can impact lifestyle choices and longevity in diverse ways across regions.

Can advancements in robotics and exoskeleton technology assist in enhancing the quality of life for the elderly and potentially impact longevity?

Robotics and exoskeletons can aid in mobility and physical activities, potentially improving the quality of life for the elderly, although their direct impact on longevity is still an area of exploration.

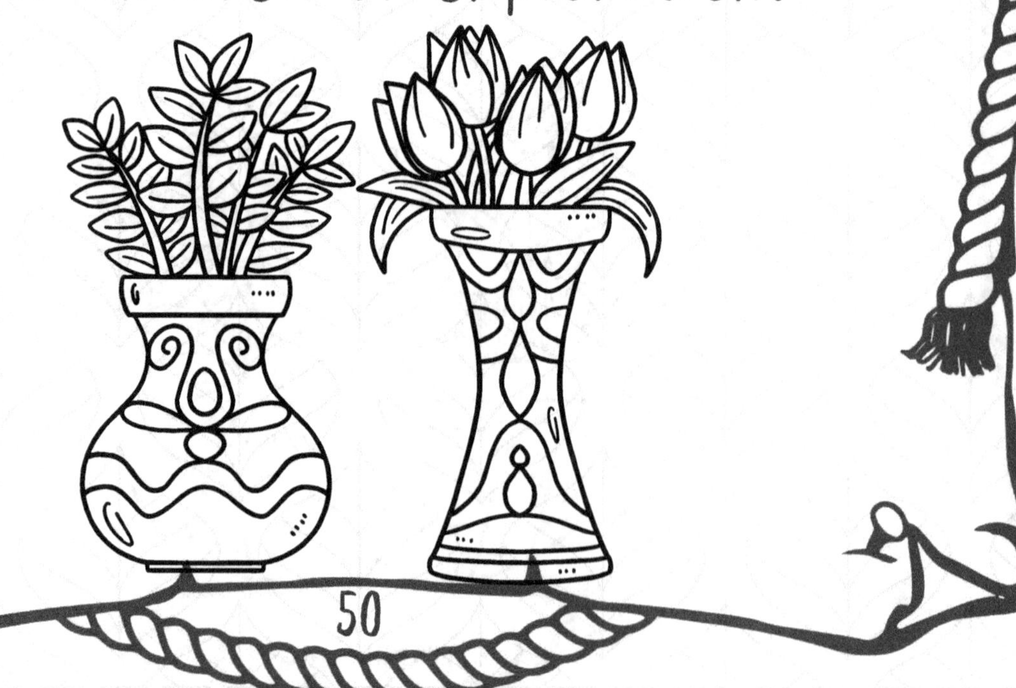

How do lifestyle practices in traditional medicine, such as Ayurveda and Traditional Chinese Medicine, relate to promoting longevity?

Traditional medicine systems often emphasize holistic approaches to health, including diet, herbal remedies, and mindfulness, which may contribute to longevity by addressing overall well-being.

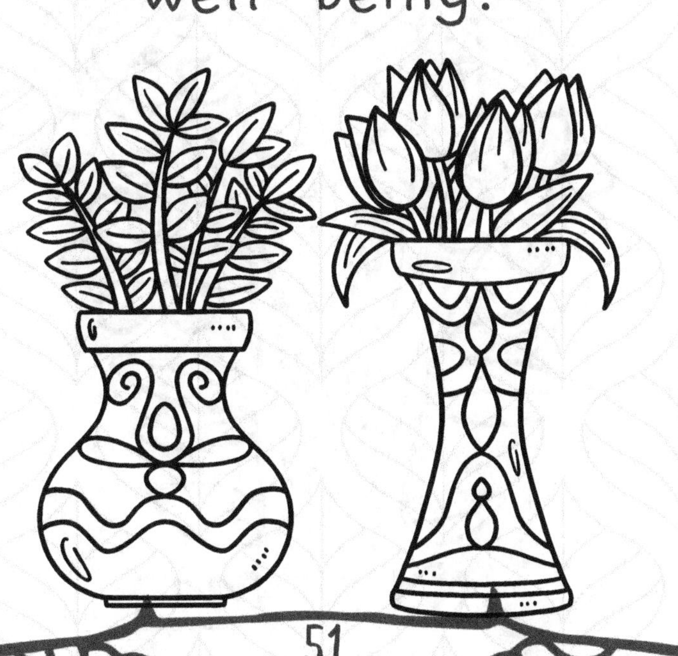

Can exposure to natural environments and green spaces positively influence longevity?

Studies suggest that spending time in nature and green spaces is associated with improved mental health and physical well-being, potentially contributing to increased longevity.

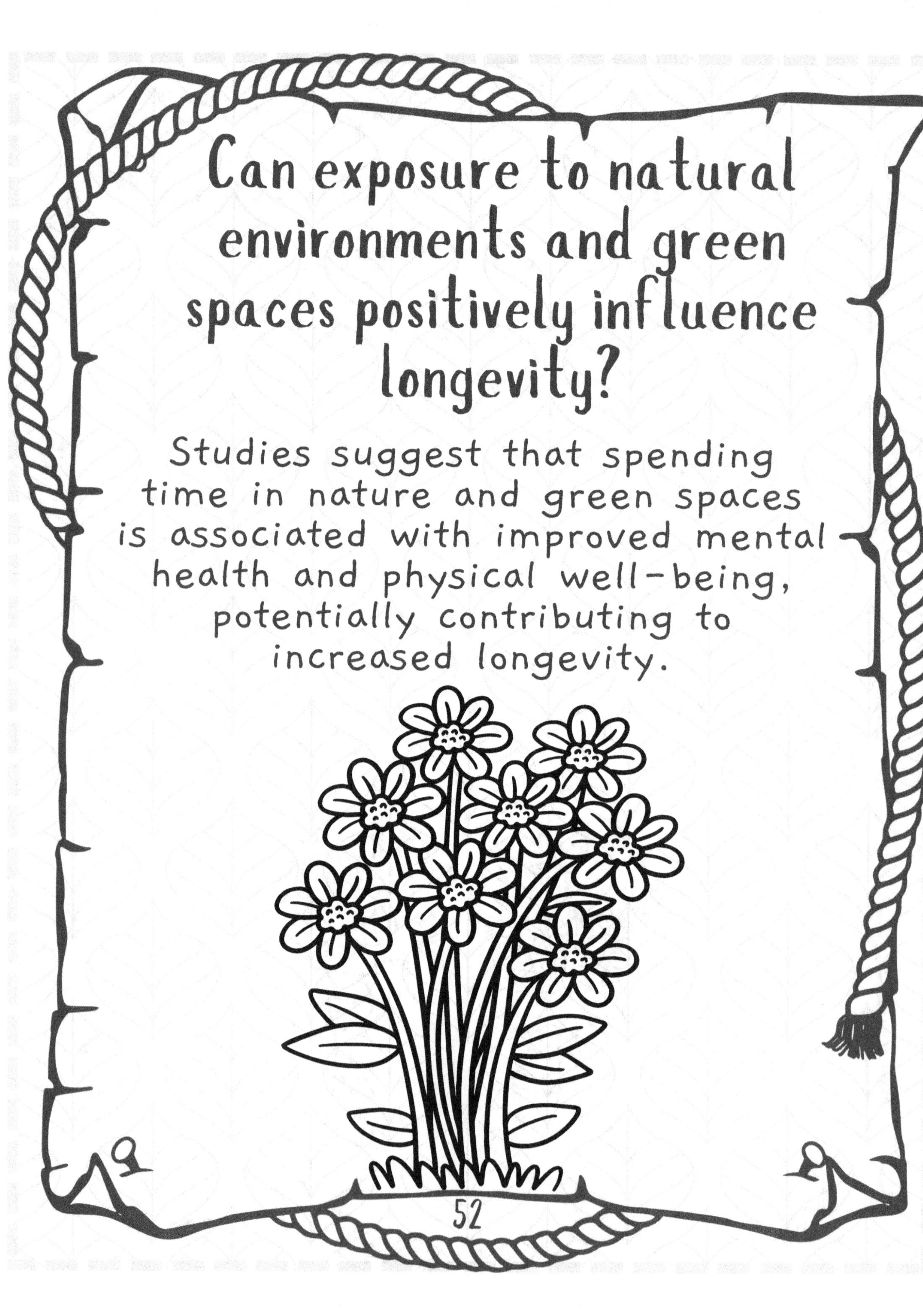

How does the microbiome-gut-brain axis relate to aging and longevity?

The intricate connection between the gut microbiome and the brain influences various aspects of health, including cognitive function, and may play a role in aging and longevity.

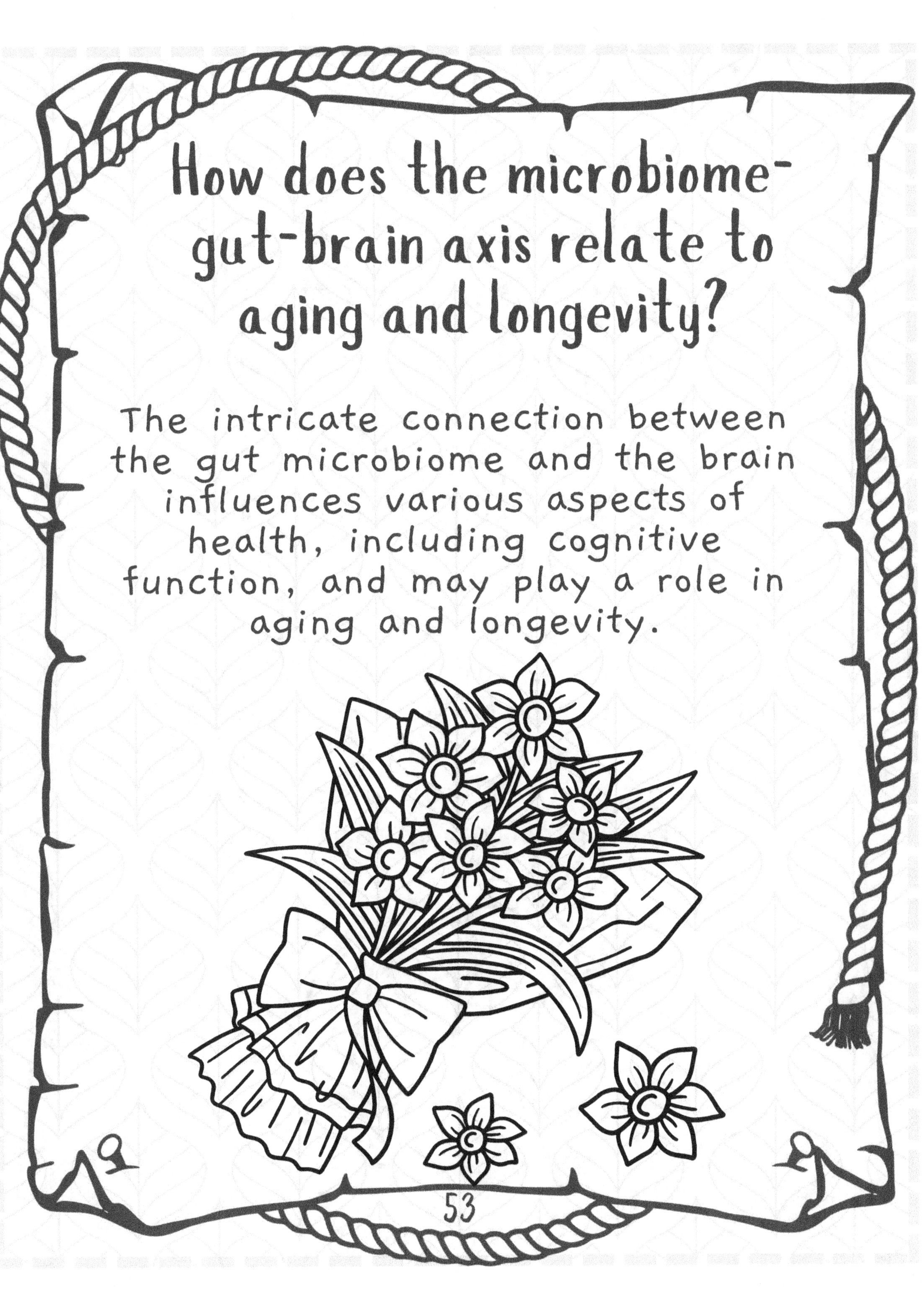

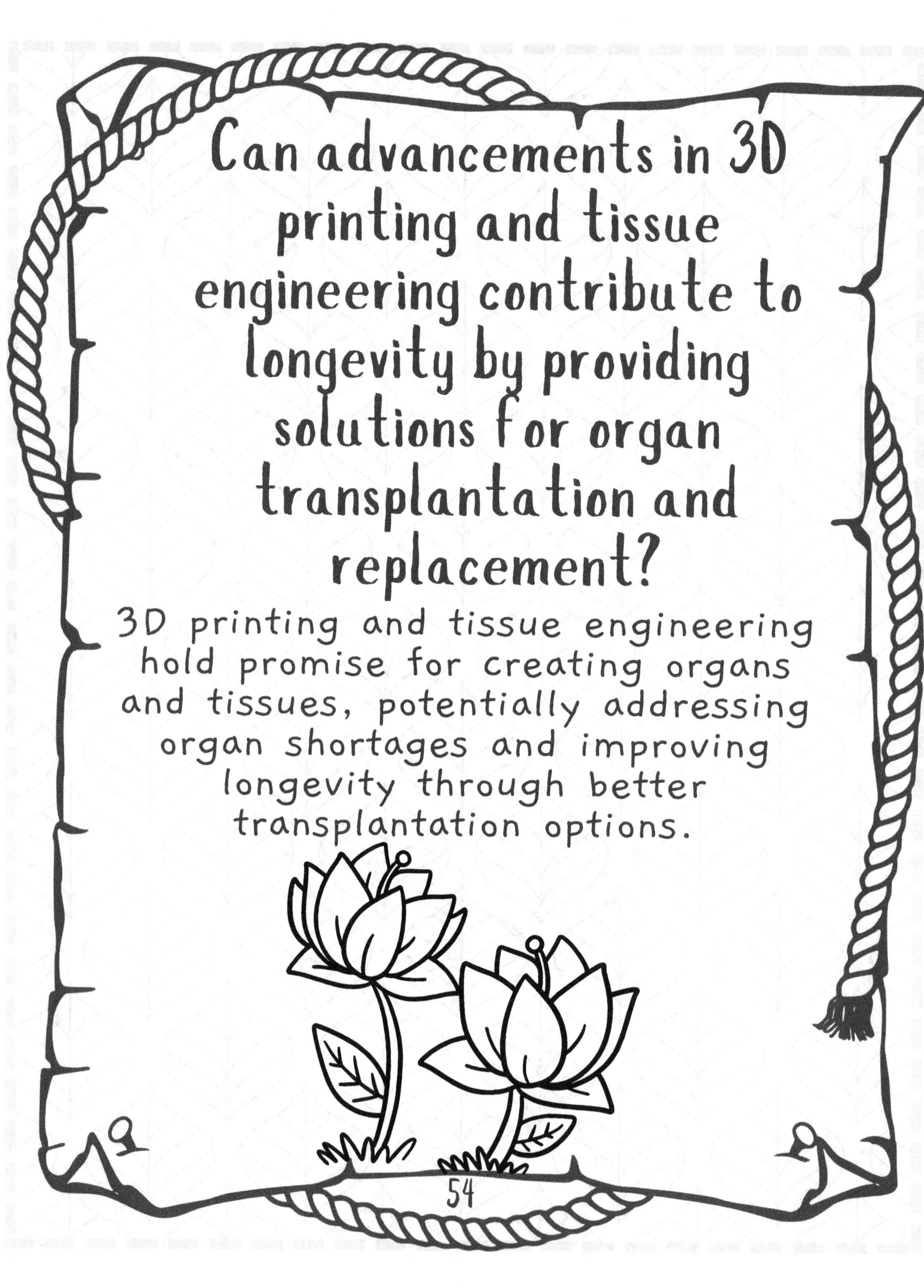

Can advancements in 3D printing and tissue engineering contribute to longevity by providing solutions for organ transplantation and replacement?

3D printing and tissue engineering hold promise for creating organs and tissues, potentially addressing organ shortages and improving longevity through better transplantation options.

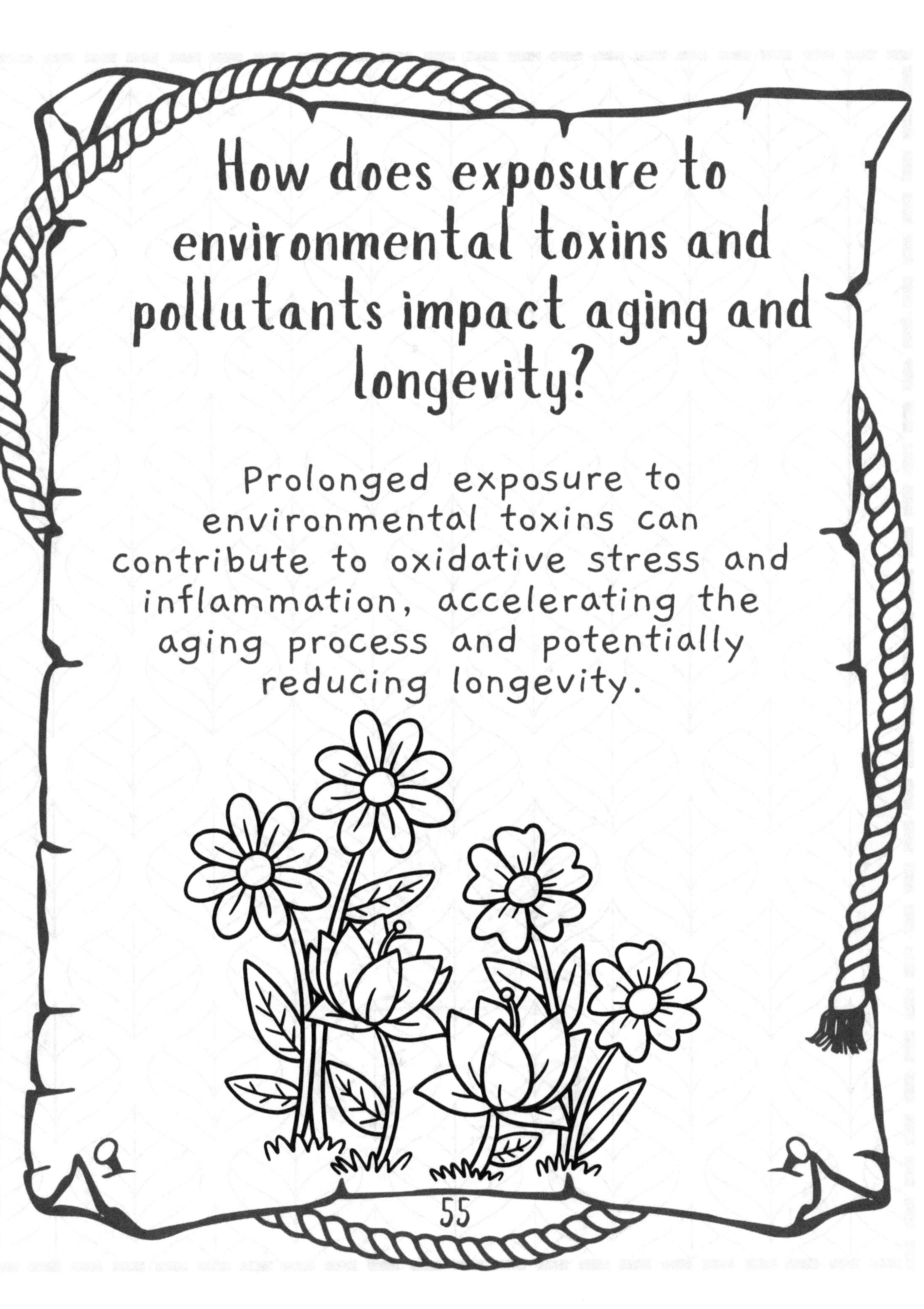

How does exposure to environmental toxins and pollutants impact aging and longevity?

Prolonged exposure to environmental toxins can contribute to oxidative stress and inflammation, accelerating the aging process and potentially reducing longevity.

Can the study of the microbiome influence dietary recommendations for promoting longevity?

Understanding how the microbiome interacts with dietary choices may lead to personalized dietary recommendations that promote a healthy gut environment and potentially impact longevity.

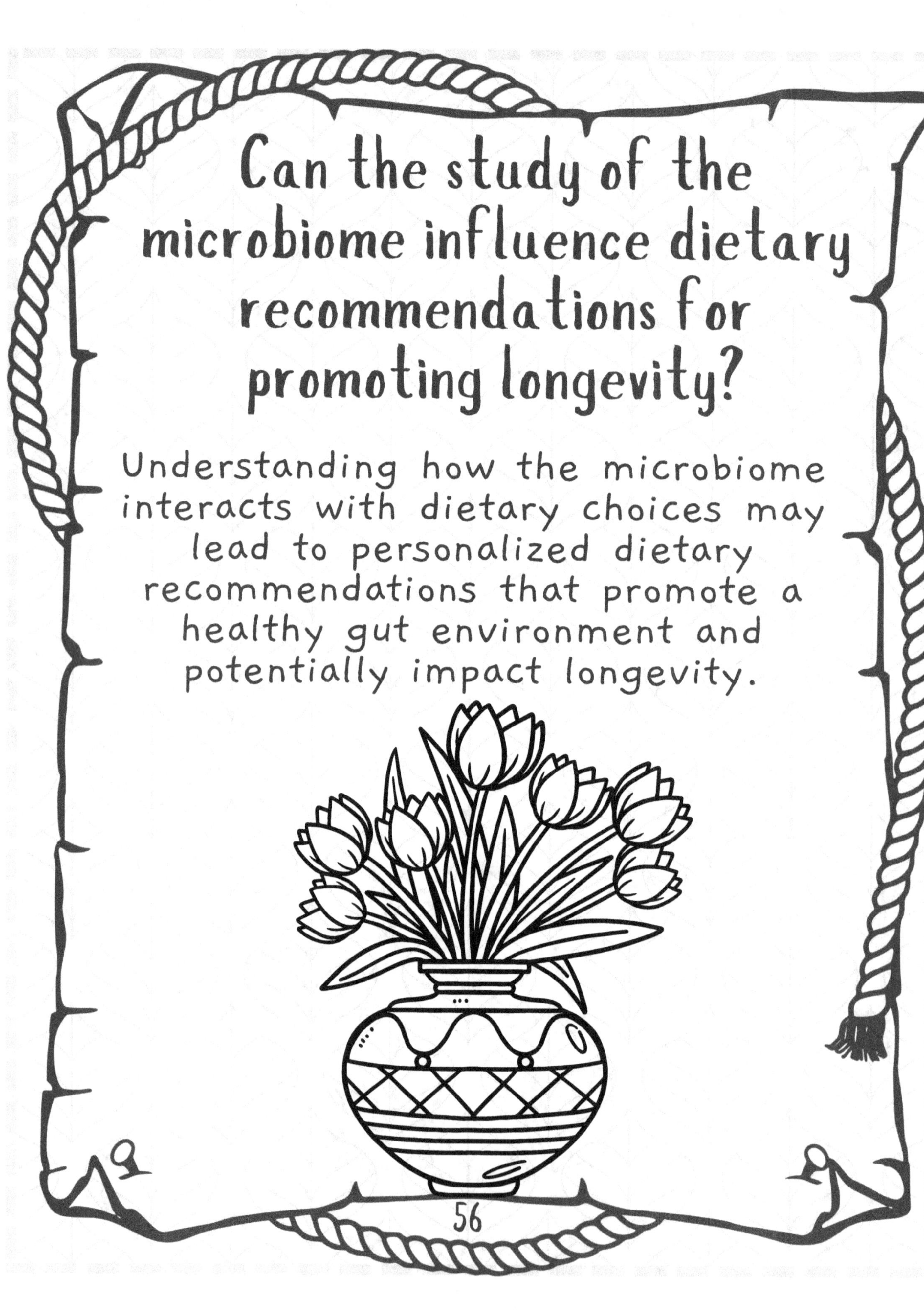

How does the interaction between genes and the environment (epigenetics) contribute to individual variations in longevity?

Epigenetic modifications resulting from the interplay between genes and the environment can contribute to individual variations in aging and longevity outcomes.

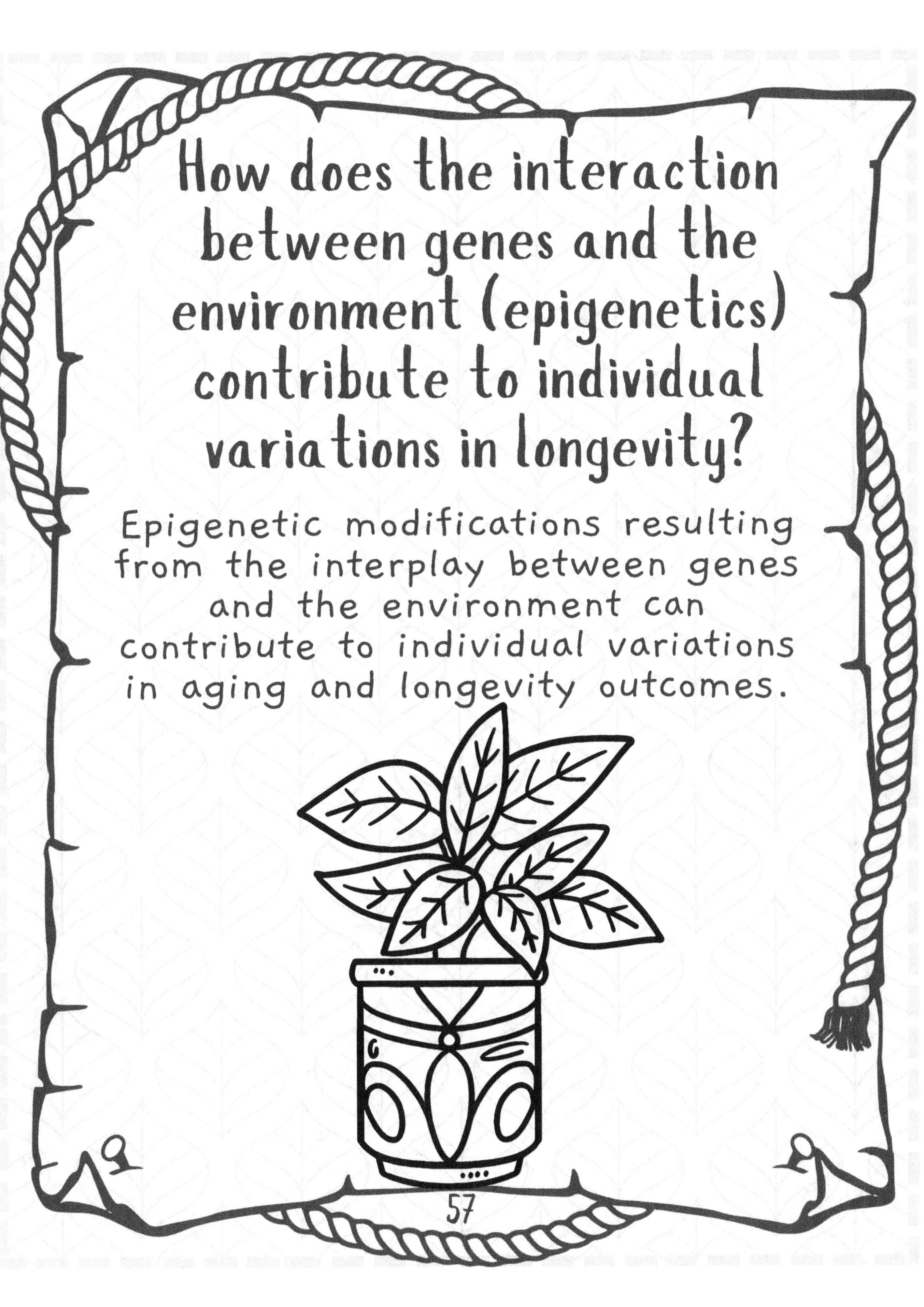

Can lifestyle interventions, such as cognitive training and mental exercises, impact cognitive longevity and reduce the risk of neurodegenerative diseases?

Cognitive training and mental exercises are being explored for their potential to maintain cognitive function, potentially influencing cognitive longevity and reducing the risk of diseases like Alzheimer's.

How do societal attitudes towards aging and the elderly influence policies related to healthcare, retirement, and overall support systems?

Societal perceptions of aging can shape policies and support systems. Positive attitudes may lead to better healthcare infrastructure and social programs, positively influencing longevity.

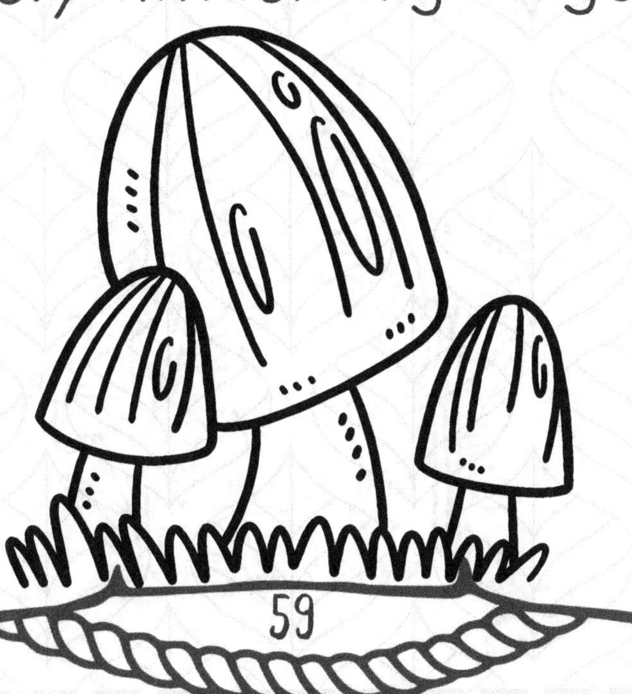

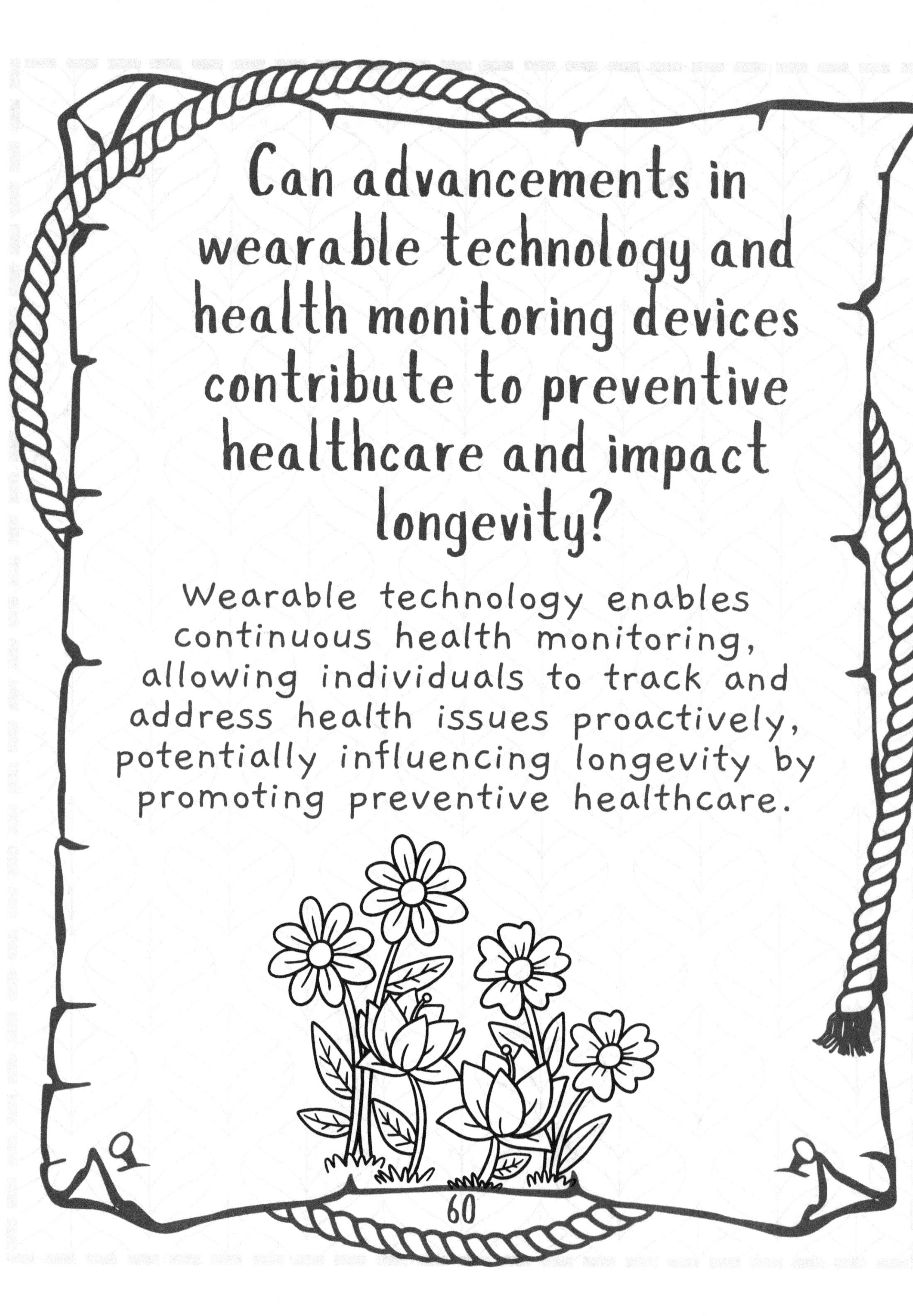

Can advancements in wearable technology and health monitoring devices contribute to preventive healthcare and impact longevity?

Wearable technology enables continuous health monitoring, allowing individuals to track and address health issues proactively, potentially influencing longevity by promoting preventive healthcare.

Balancing individual freedoms with public health measures can impact the spread of diseases and overall health outcomes, influencing longevity in diverse societal contexts.

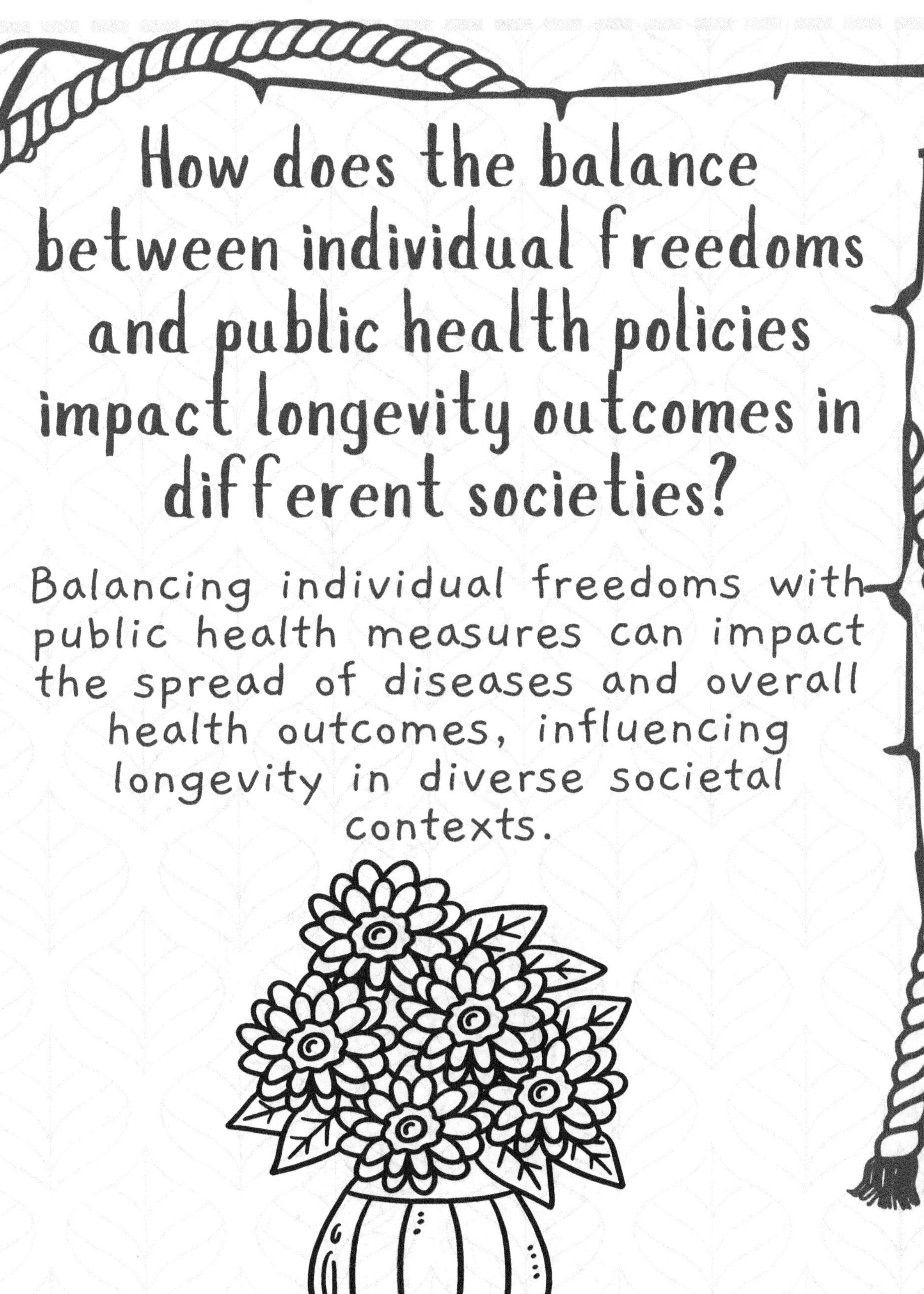

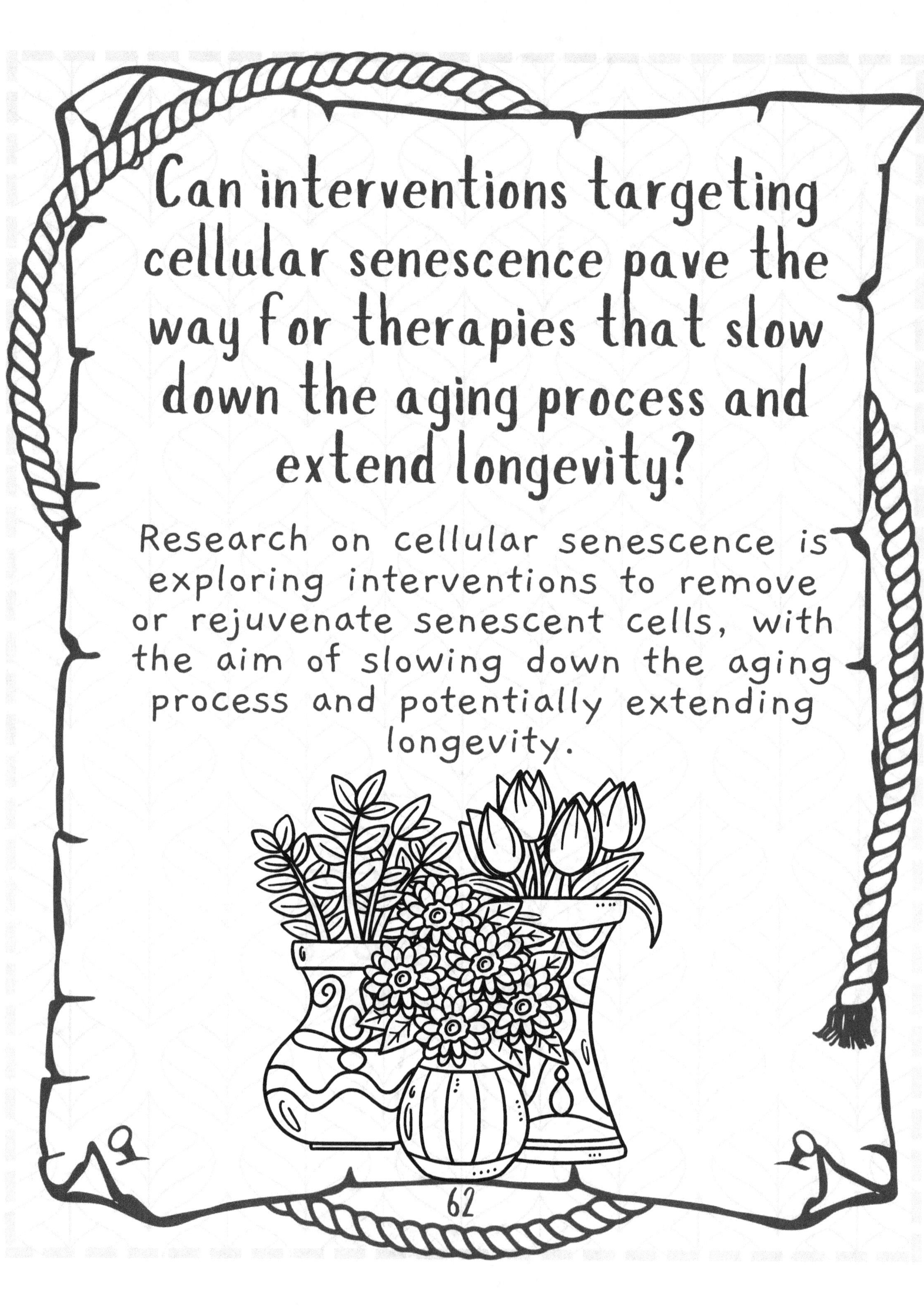

Can interventions targeting cellular senescence pave the way for therapies that slow down the aging process and extend longevity?

Research on cellular senescence is exploring interventions to remove or rejuvenate senescent cells, with the aim of slowing down the aging process and potentially extending longevity.

How does access to education about healthy aging impact lifestyle choices and longevity in various demographic groups?

Access to education about healthy aging can empower individuals to make informed lifestyle choices, potentially positively impacting longevity across diverse demographic groups.

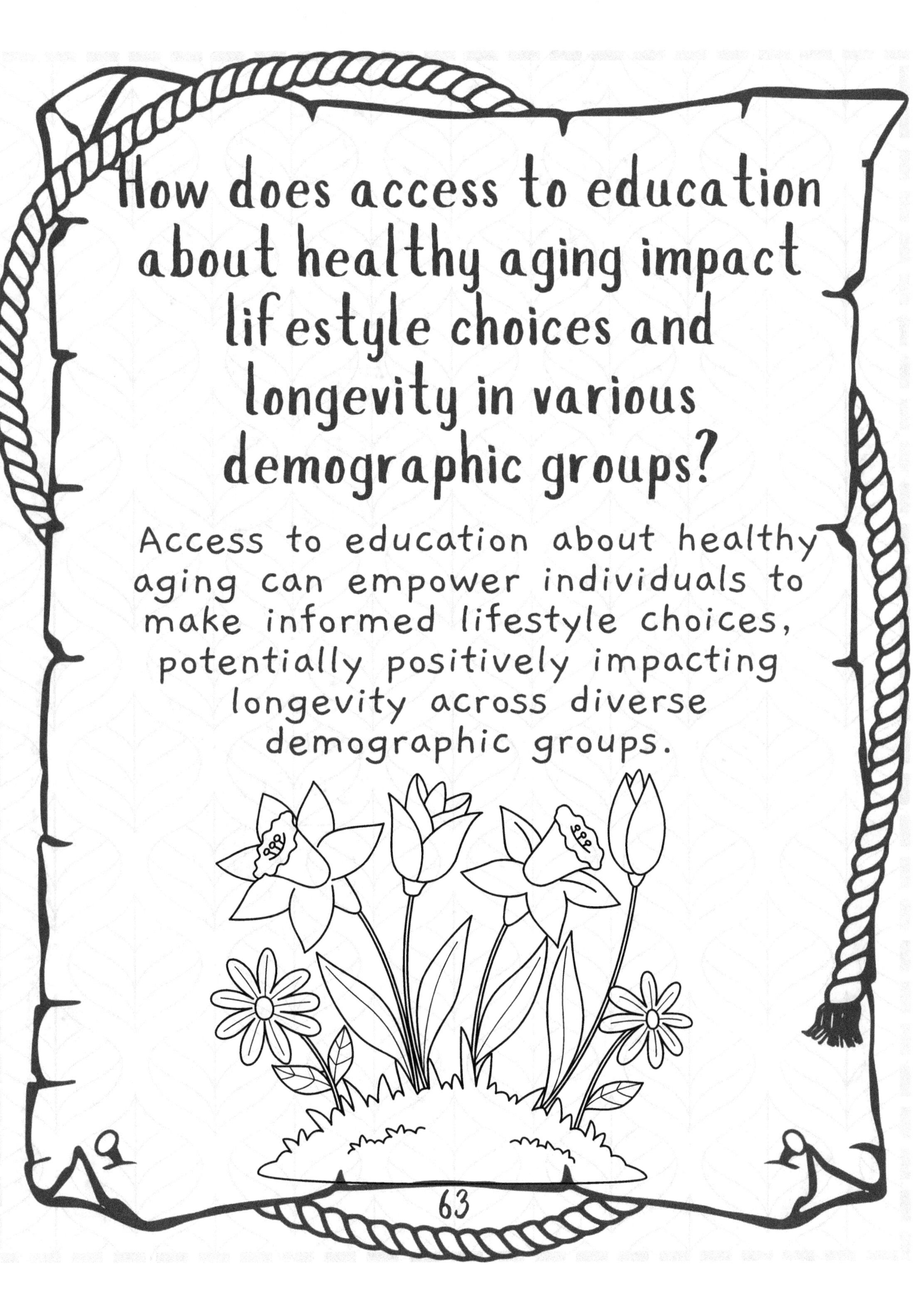

Can personalized medicine and genetic testing help individuals make lifestyle choices that align with their genetic predispositions for better longevity outcomes?

Personalized medicine and genetic testing may provide insights into individual health risks, enabling targeted lifestyle choices that align with genetic predispositions for improved longevity.

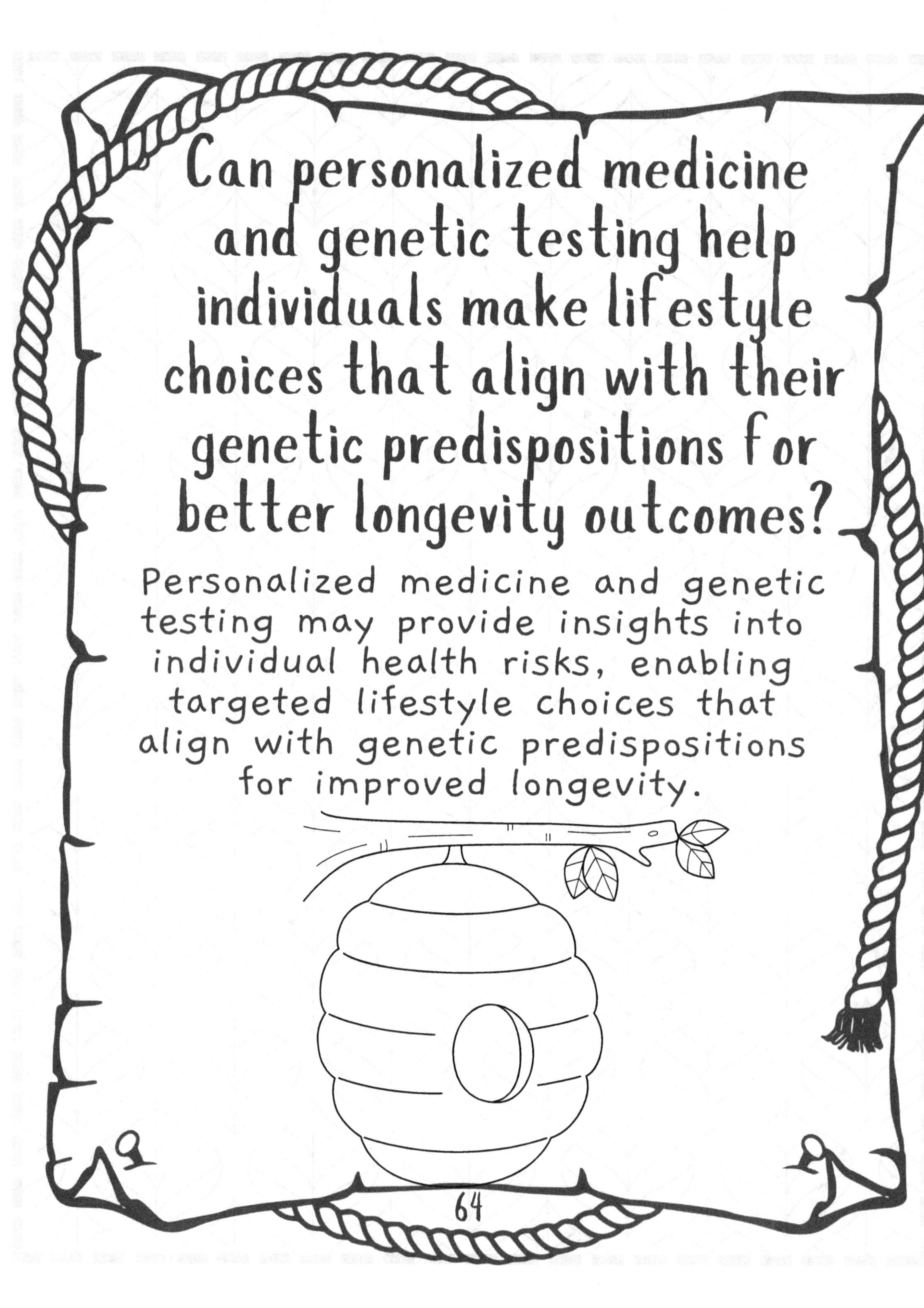

How does the role of social and emotional support impact the mental and emotional well-being of individuals, potentially contributing to longevity?

Social and emotional support systems are crucial for mental health. Strong social connections may positively influence emotional well-being and contribute to increased longevity.

Can community-based interventions and public health campaigns promote healthier lifestyles and positively impact longevity at the population level?

Community-based interventions and public health campaigns play a vital role in raising awareness and promoting healthier lifestyles, potentially influencing longevity on a larger scale.

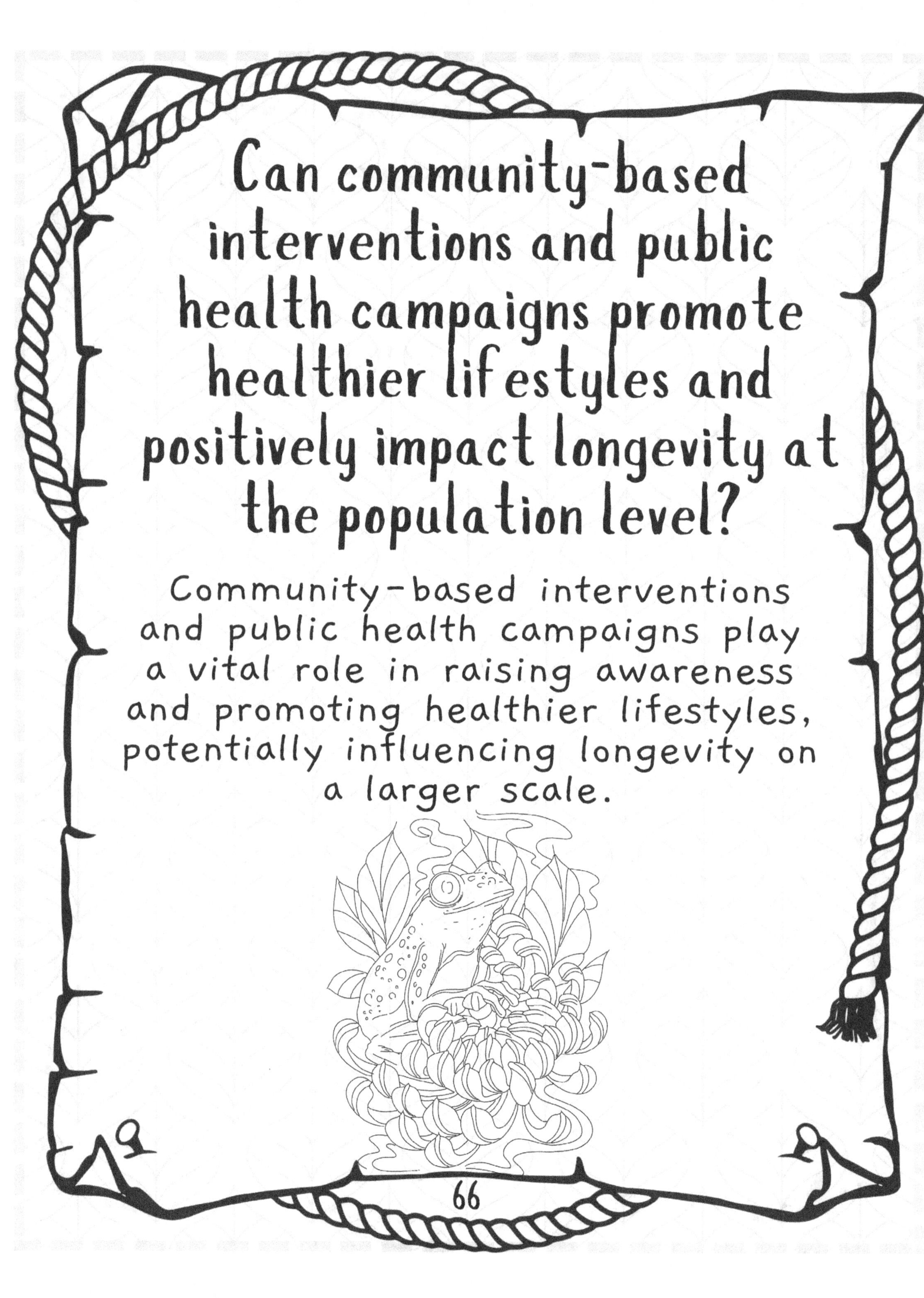

How do emerging technologies like virtual reality contribute to mental and physical well-being in older populations, potentially impacting longevity?

Virtual reality technologies offer opportunities for cognitive and physical engagement, potentially enhancing the overall well-being of older individuals and contributing to longevity.

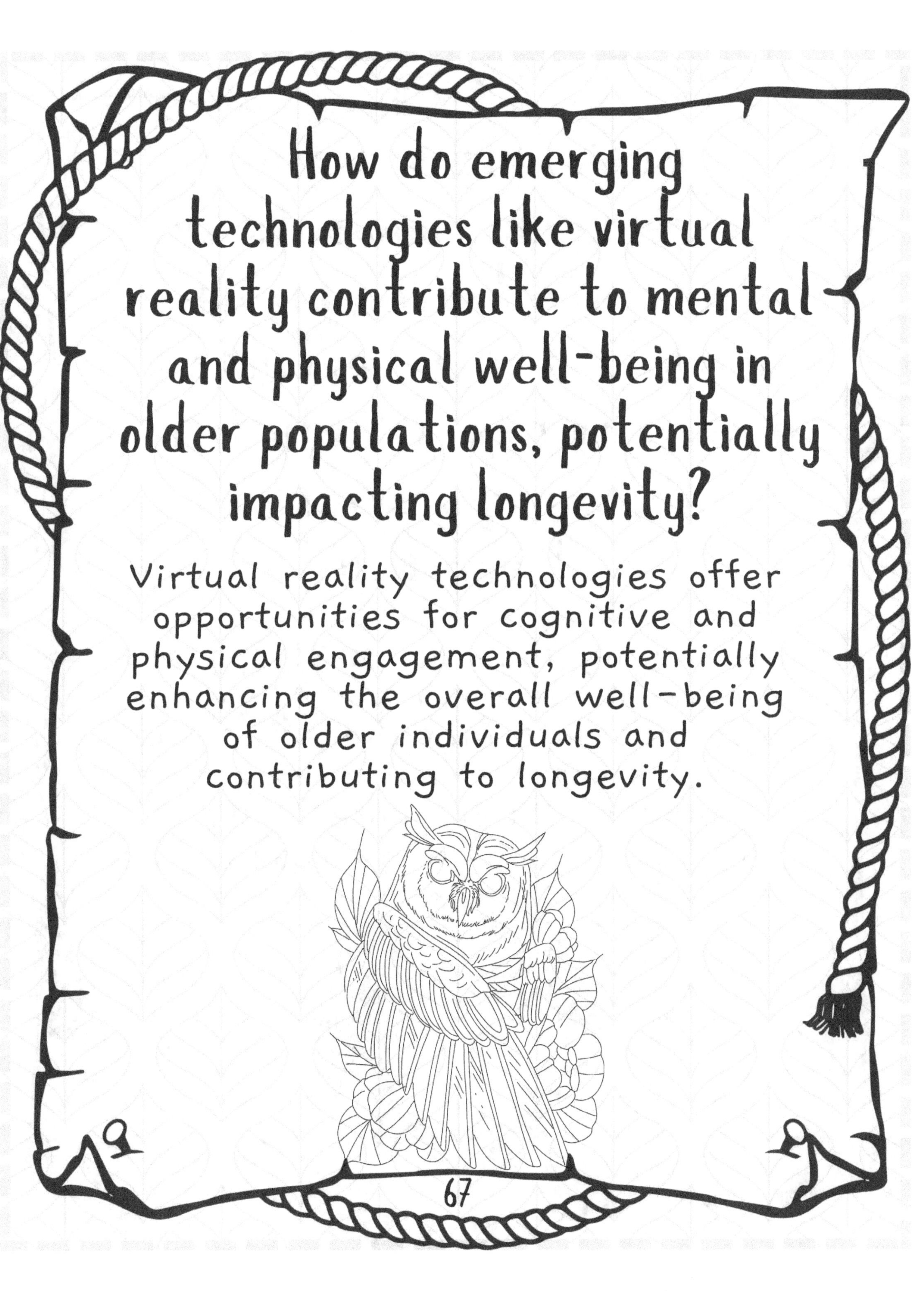

an the exploration of extreme environments, such as space travel, provide insights into the effects of microgravity and radiation on the aging process and longevity?

Studying the impact of space travel on the human body may offer insights into the effects of unique stressors like microgravity and radiation, potentially influencing longevity research.

How do economic incentives for healthy behaviors and preventive healthcare impact individual choices and contribute to longevity?

Economic incentives, such as reduced insurance premiums for healthy behaviors, may encourage individuals to adopt healthier lifestyles, positively impacting longevity outcomes.

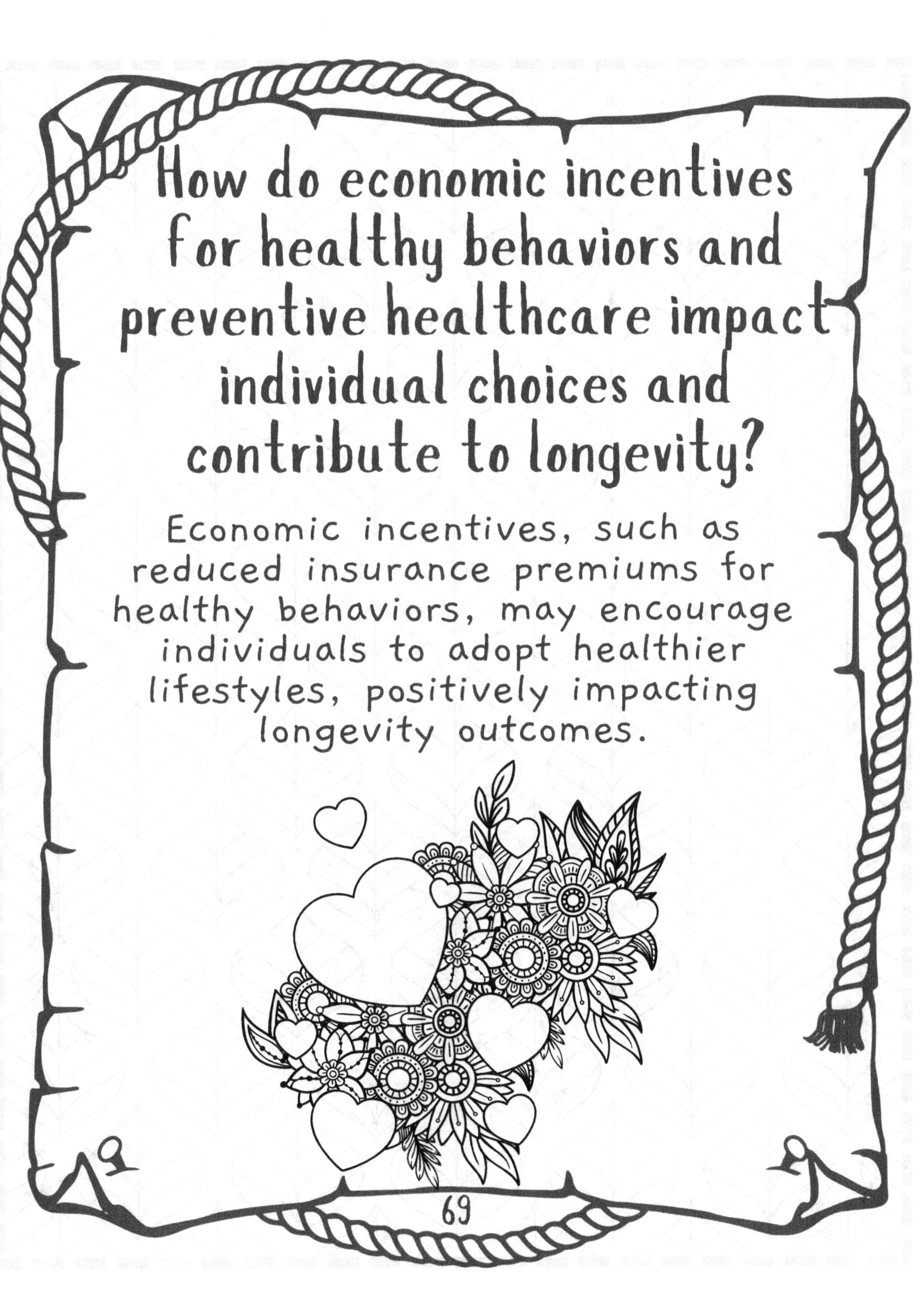

Can interventions targeting mitochondrial health and function impact the aging process and contribute to increased longevity?

Mitochondria play a crucial role in cellular energy production. Research on interventions to maintain mitochondrial health may influence the aging process and longevity.

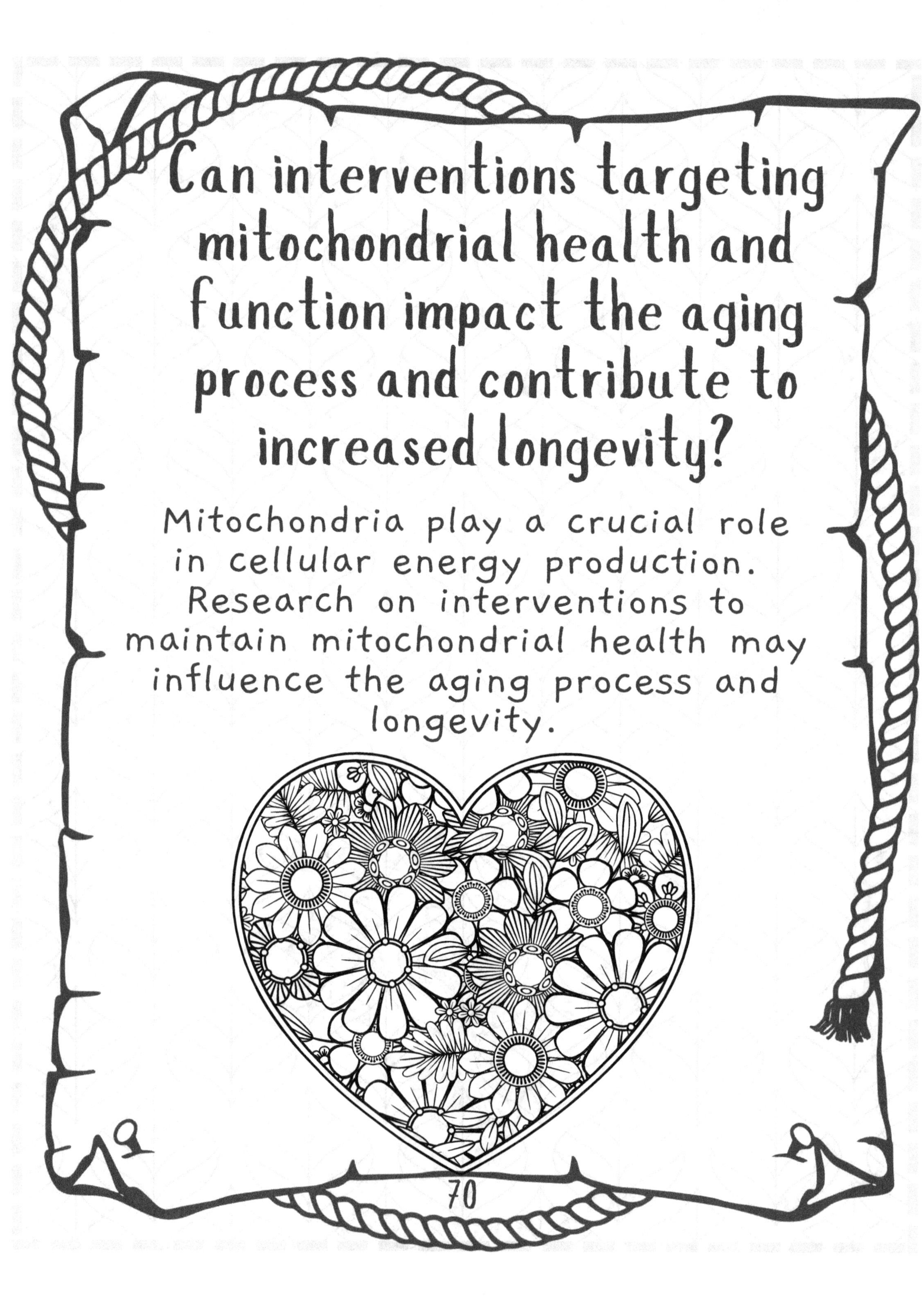

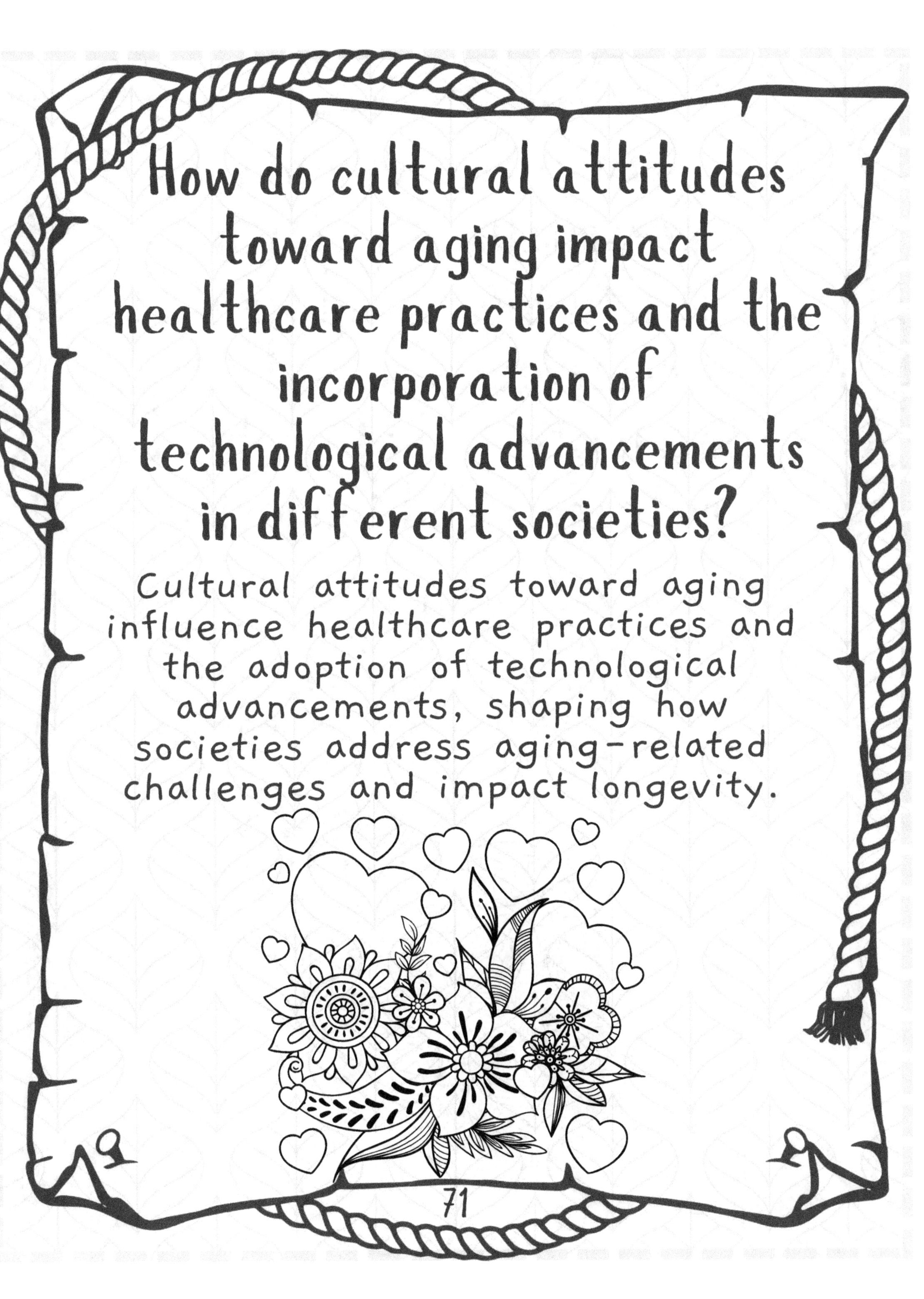

How do cultural attitudes toward aging impact healthcare practices and the incorporation of technological advancements in different societies?

Cultural attitudes toward aging influence healthcare practices and the adoption of technological advancements, shaping how societies address aging-related challenges and impact longevity.

Can advancements in personalized nutrition, considering an individual's unique genetic makeup, contribute to better health outcomes and longevity?

Personalized nutrition, tailored to an individual's genetic profile, may optimize dietary choices for improved health and potentially impact longevity.

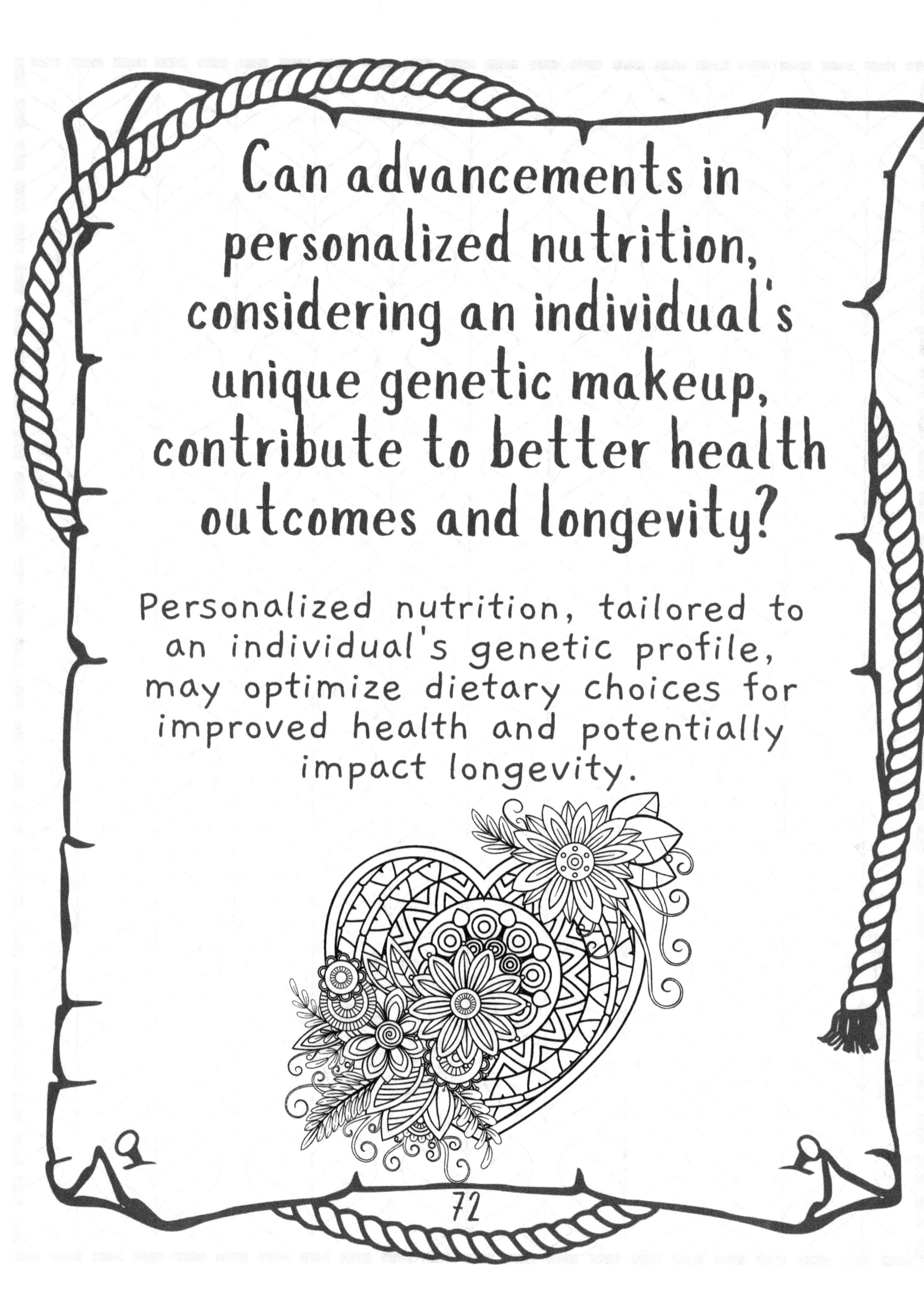

How does the accessibility and affordability of healthcare services influence health outcomes and longevity in different regions?

Unequal access to healthcare services can contribute to disparities in health outcomes, affecting longevity. Addressing healthcare accessibility is crucial for improving longevity globally.

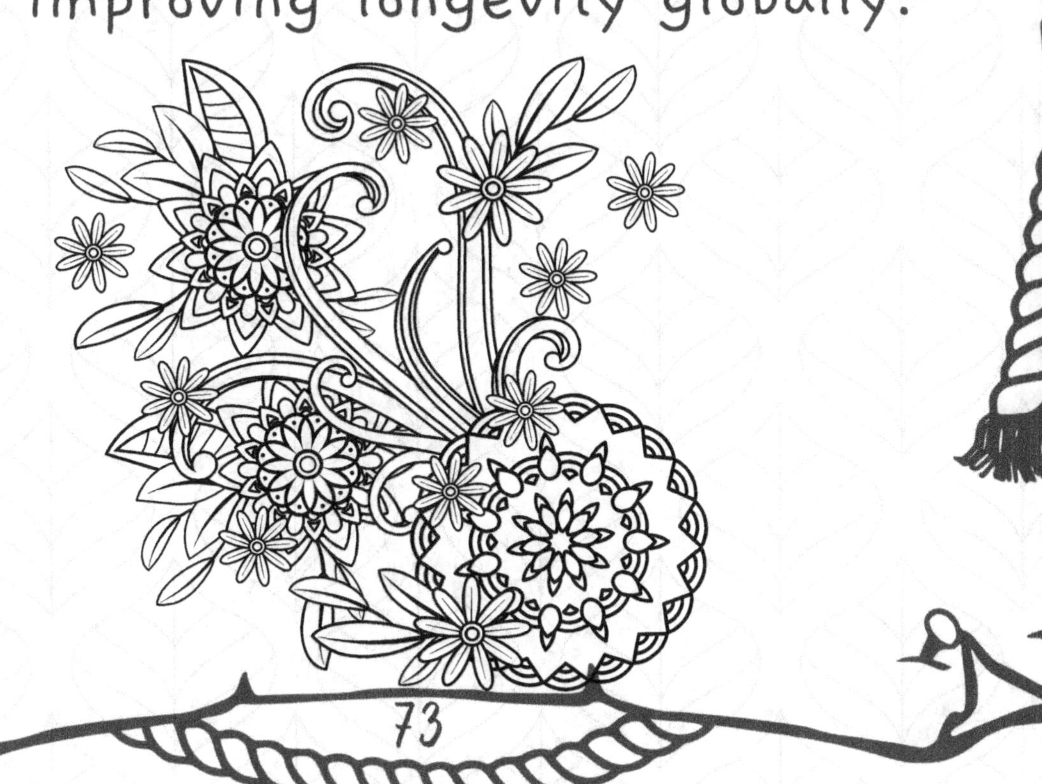

How do environmental conservation efforts impact the quality of air, water, and food, and subsequently influence health and longevity?

Environmental conservation efforts contribute to improved air and water quality, positively impacting public health and potentially influencing longevity.

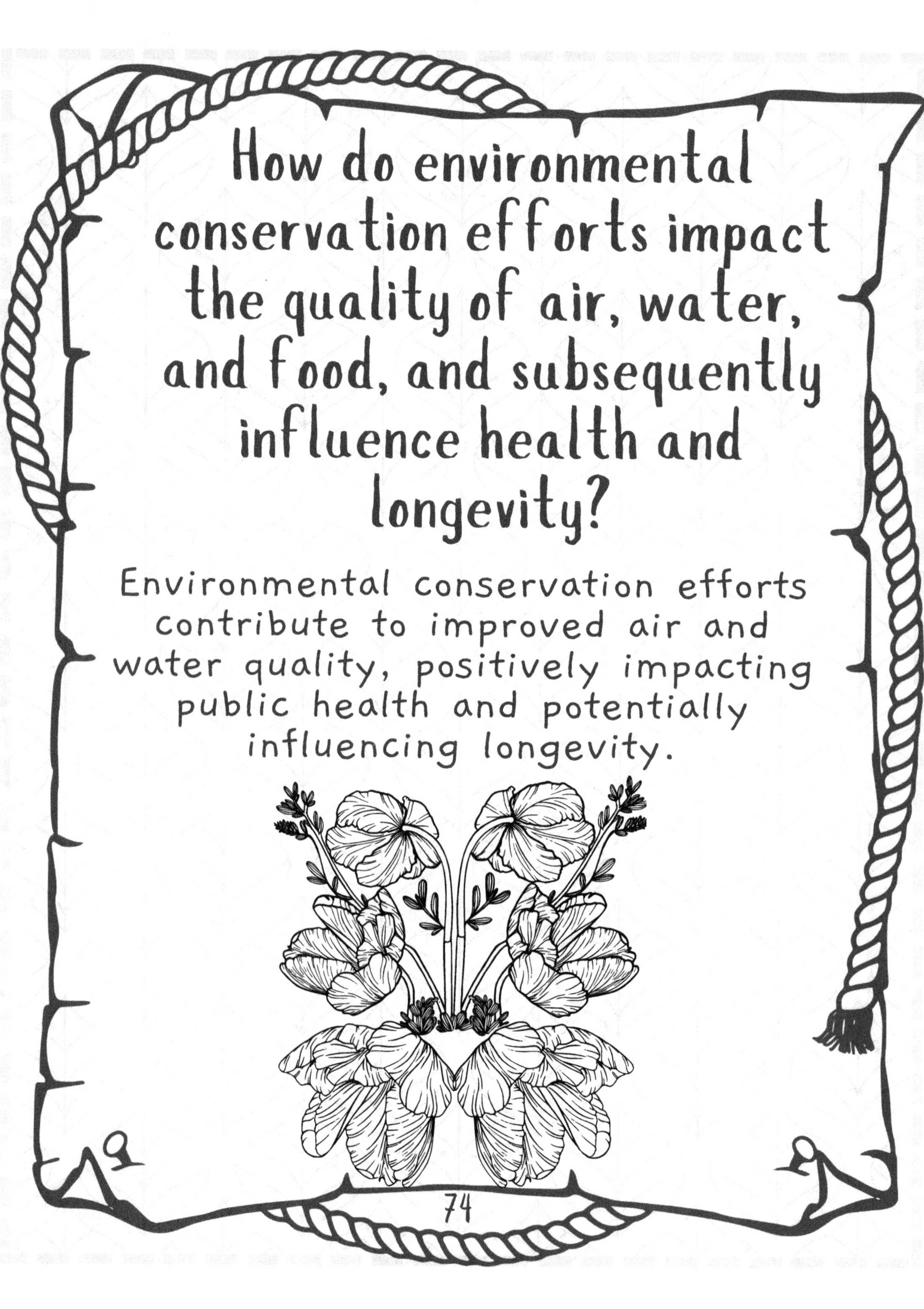

Can the study of neuroplasticity and brain training exercises contribute to maintaining cognitive function and longevity in aging populations?

Neuroplasticity research and brain training exercises aim to maintain cognitive function in aging individuals, potentially impacting longevity by addressing age-related cognitive decline.

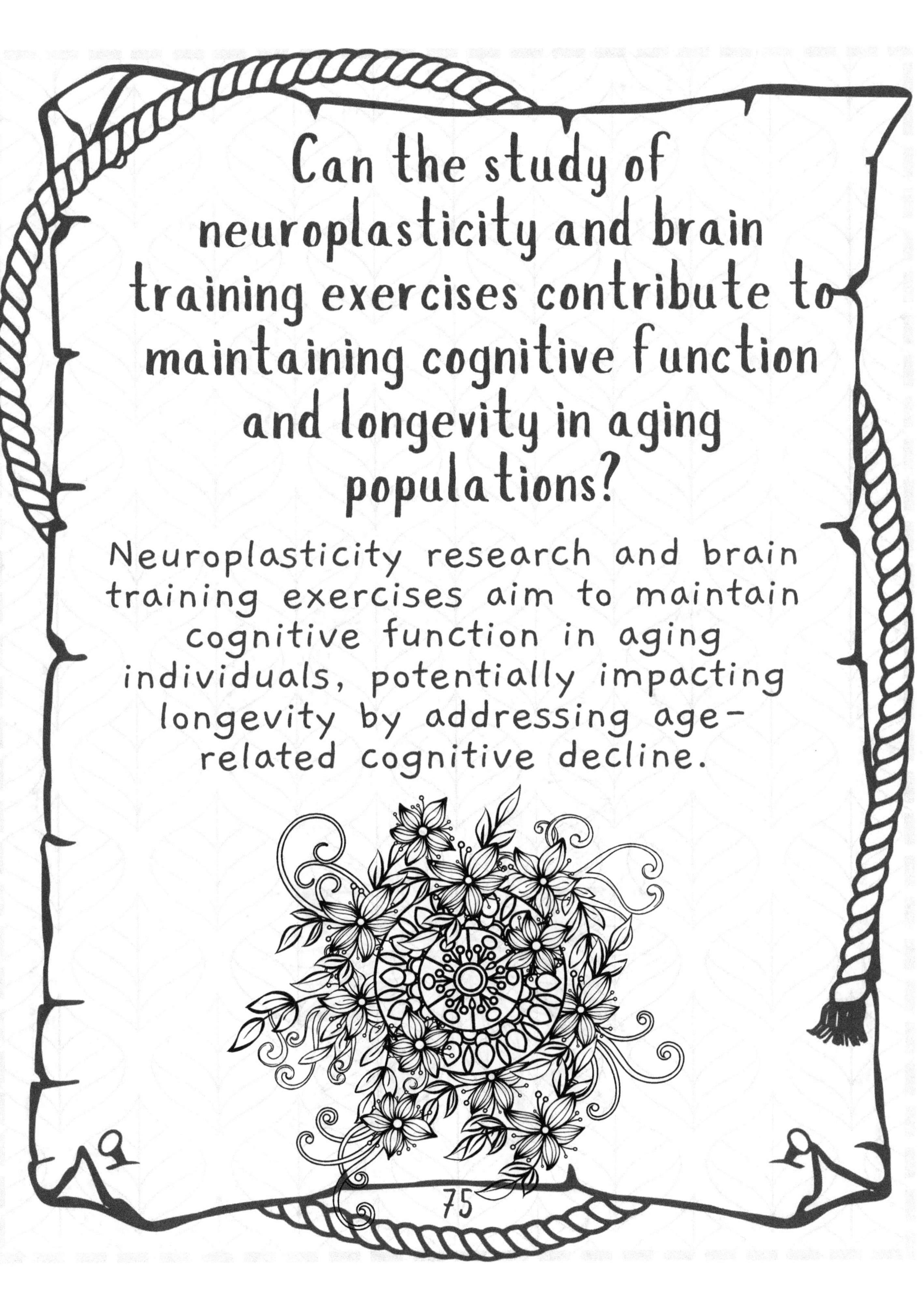

How do economic recessions and financial instability impact health outcomes and potentially influence longevity in affected populations?

Economic downturns can lead to increased stress and reduced access to healthcare, potentially impacting health outcomes and longevity in populations experiencing financial instability.

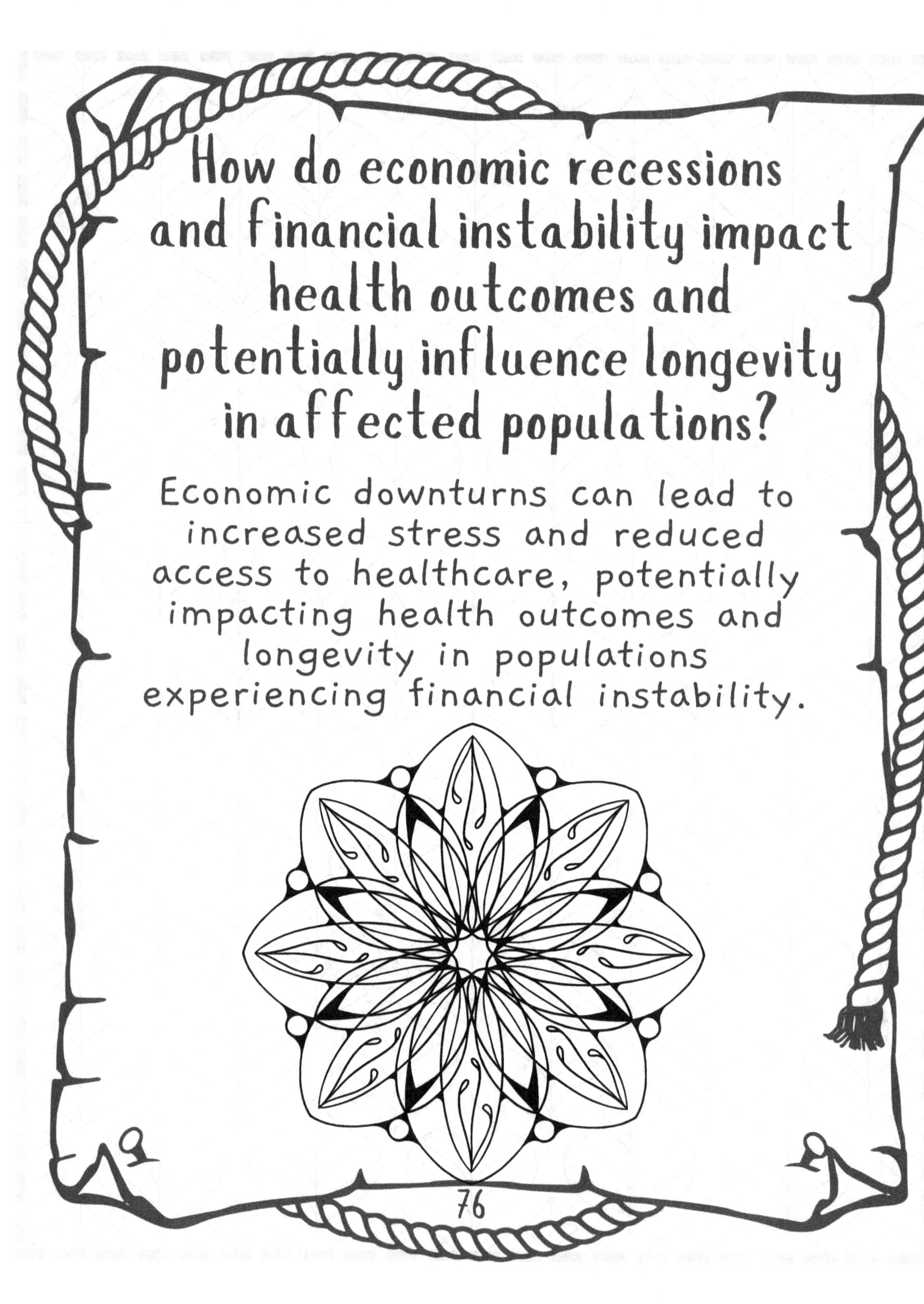

Can the integration of traditional knowledge and practices from indigenous cultures contribute to holistic approaches to health and longevity?

Incorporating traditional knowledge may provide holistic approaches to health, incorporating cultural practices that positively influence longevity and well-being.

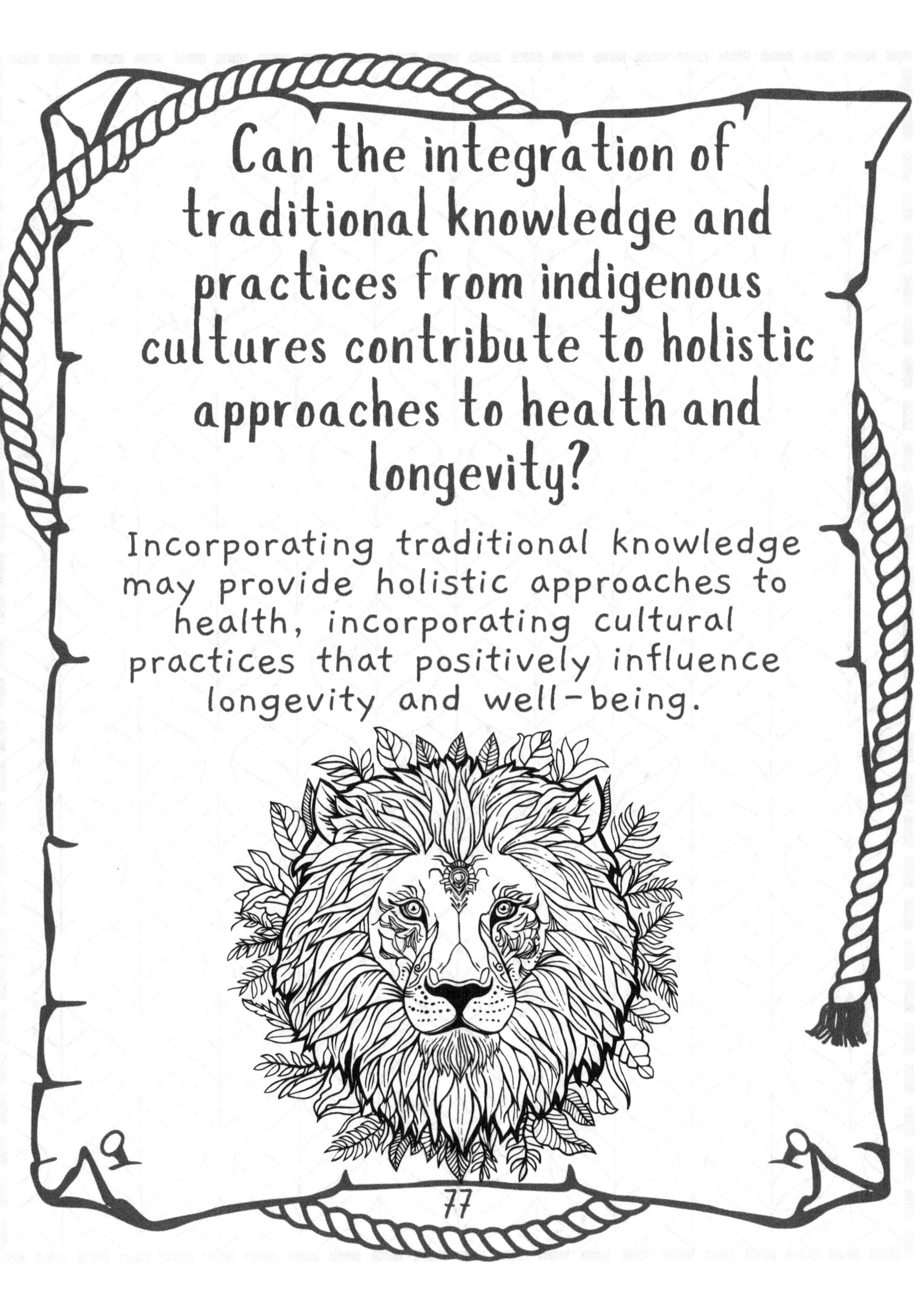

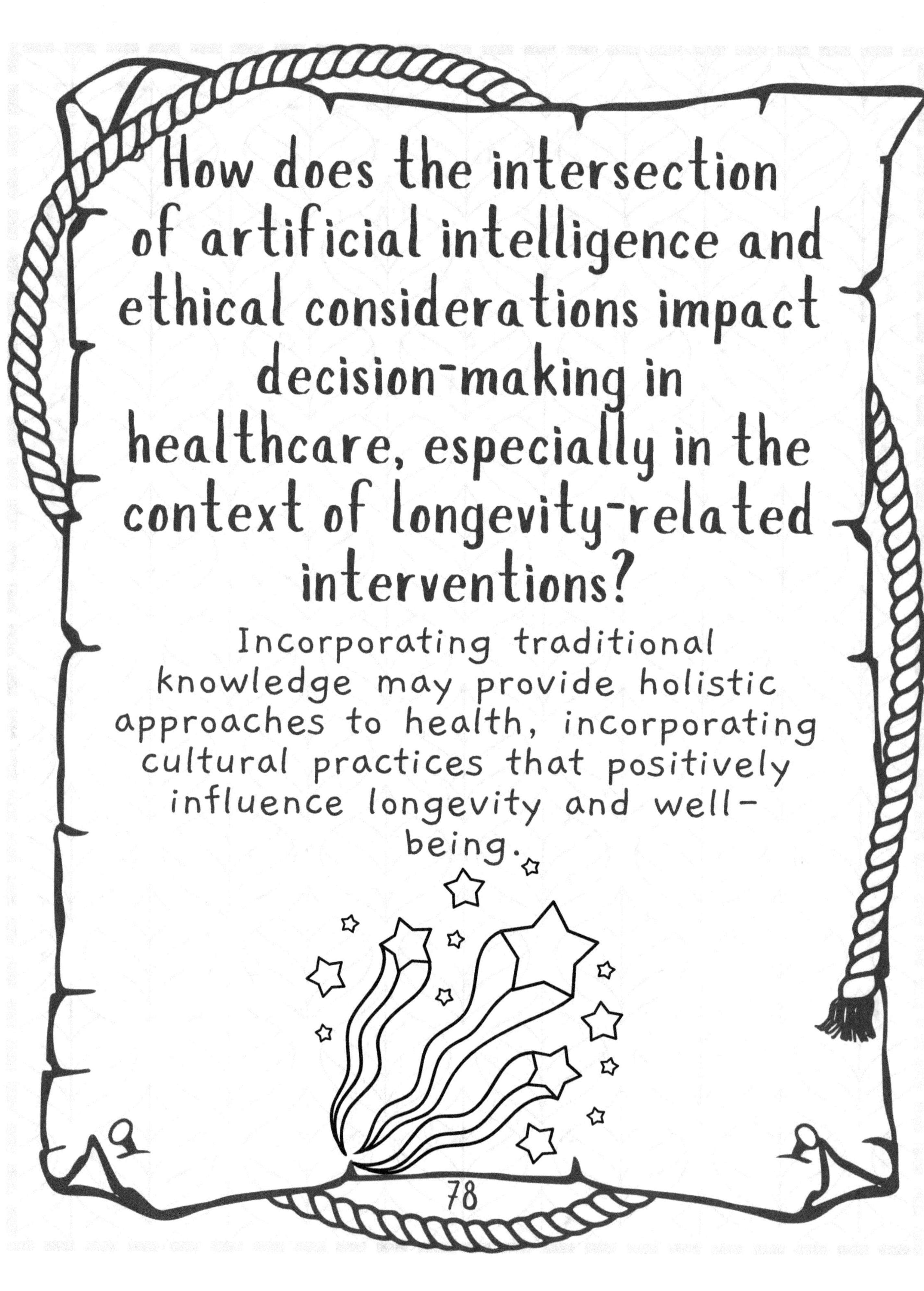

How does the intersection of artificial intelligence and ethical considerations impact decision-making in healthcare, especially in the context of longevity-related interventions?

Incorporating traditional knowledge may provide holistic approaches to health, incorporating cultural practices that positively influence longevity and well-being.

How does the intersection of artificial intelligence and ethical considerations impact decision-making in healthcare, especially in the context of longevity-related interventions?

The ethical considerations surrounding AI in healthcare, such as privacy and equity, influence decision-making, shaping how longevity-related interventions are implemented responsibly.

Can the exploration of the gut-brain axis lead to interventions that enhance mental well-being and potentially impact longevity?

Understanding the intricate relationship between the gut and the brain may lead to interventions that promote mental well-being, potentially contributing to increased longevity.

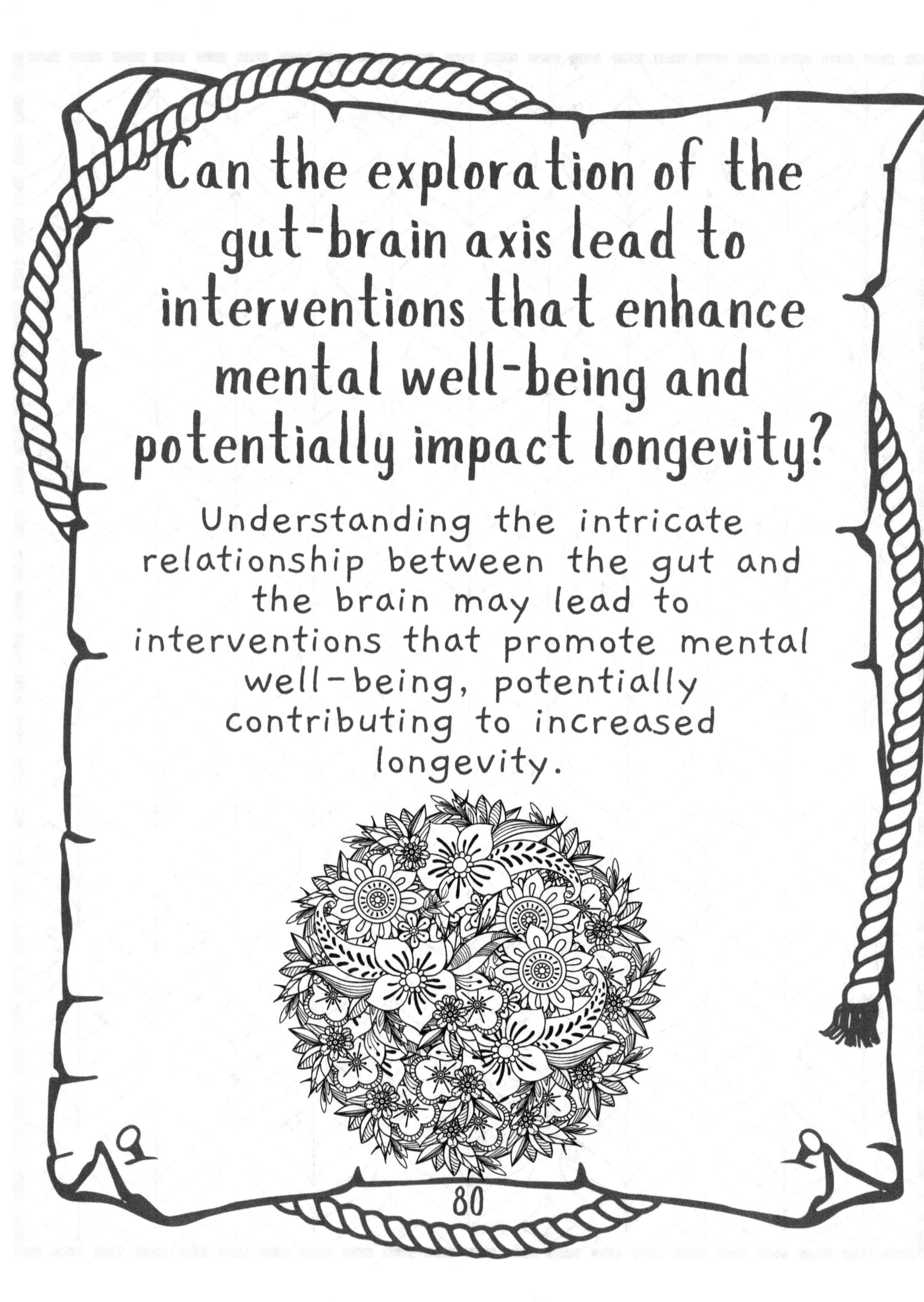

How do sleep patterns and circadian rhythm disruptions influence the risk of age-related diseases and impact longevity?

Disruptions in sleep patterns and circadian rhythms are associated with increased risks of various diseases. Maintaining healthy sleep patterns may positively influence longevity.

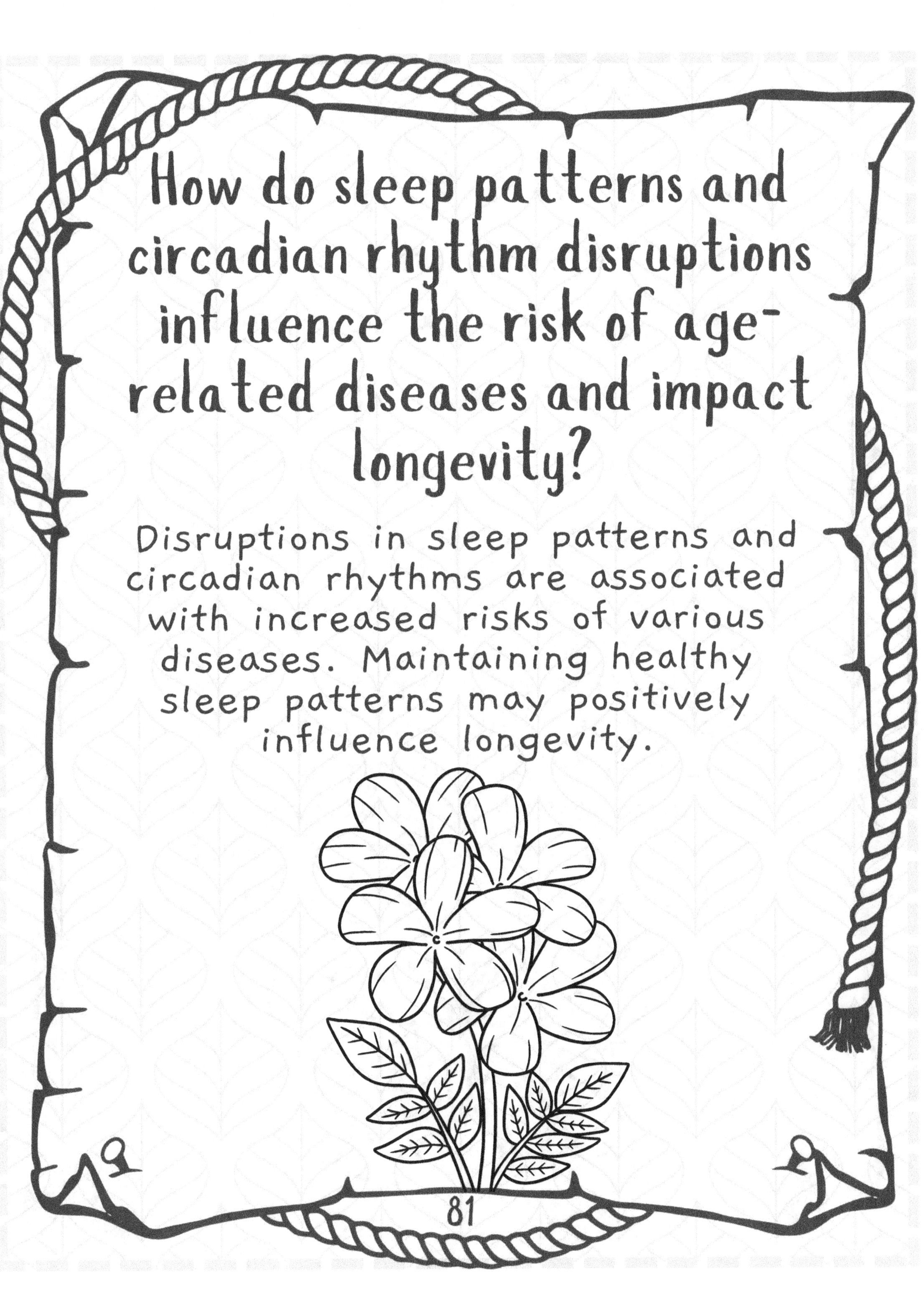

Can social entrepreneurship and innovative community initiatives contribute to addressing health disparities and promoting longevity in underserved populations?

Social entrepreneurship and community initiatives have the potential to address health disparities, improving access to resources and healthcare in underserved populations and positively impacting longevity.

How does the built environment, including urban planning and infrastructure, influence physical activity, air quality, and overall health outcomes, potentially affecting longevity?

Urban planning and infrastructure design can impact physical activity levels, air quality, and overall health. A well-designed built environment may contribute to increased longevity.

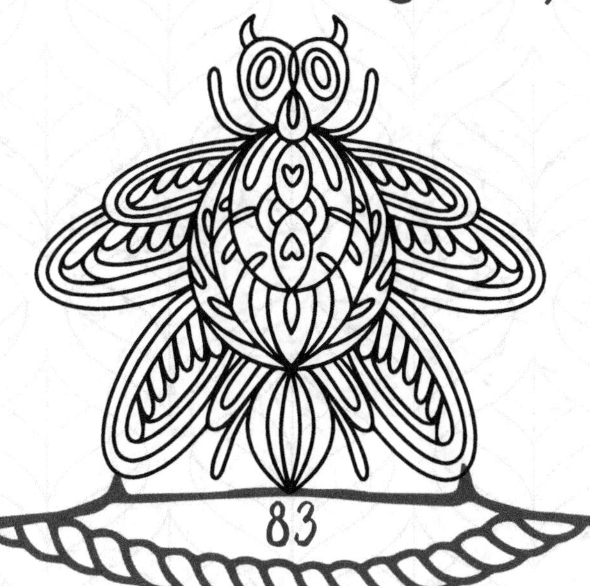

Can the study of autophagy, the cellular process of self-cleaning, provide insights into mechanisms that promote cellular health and impact longevity?

Autophagy is crucial for cellular health. Research in this area may uncover interventions that enhance autophagic processes, potentially influencing longevity.

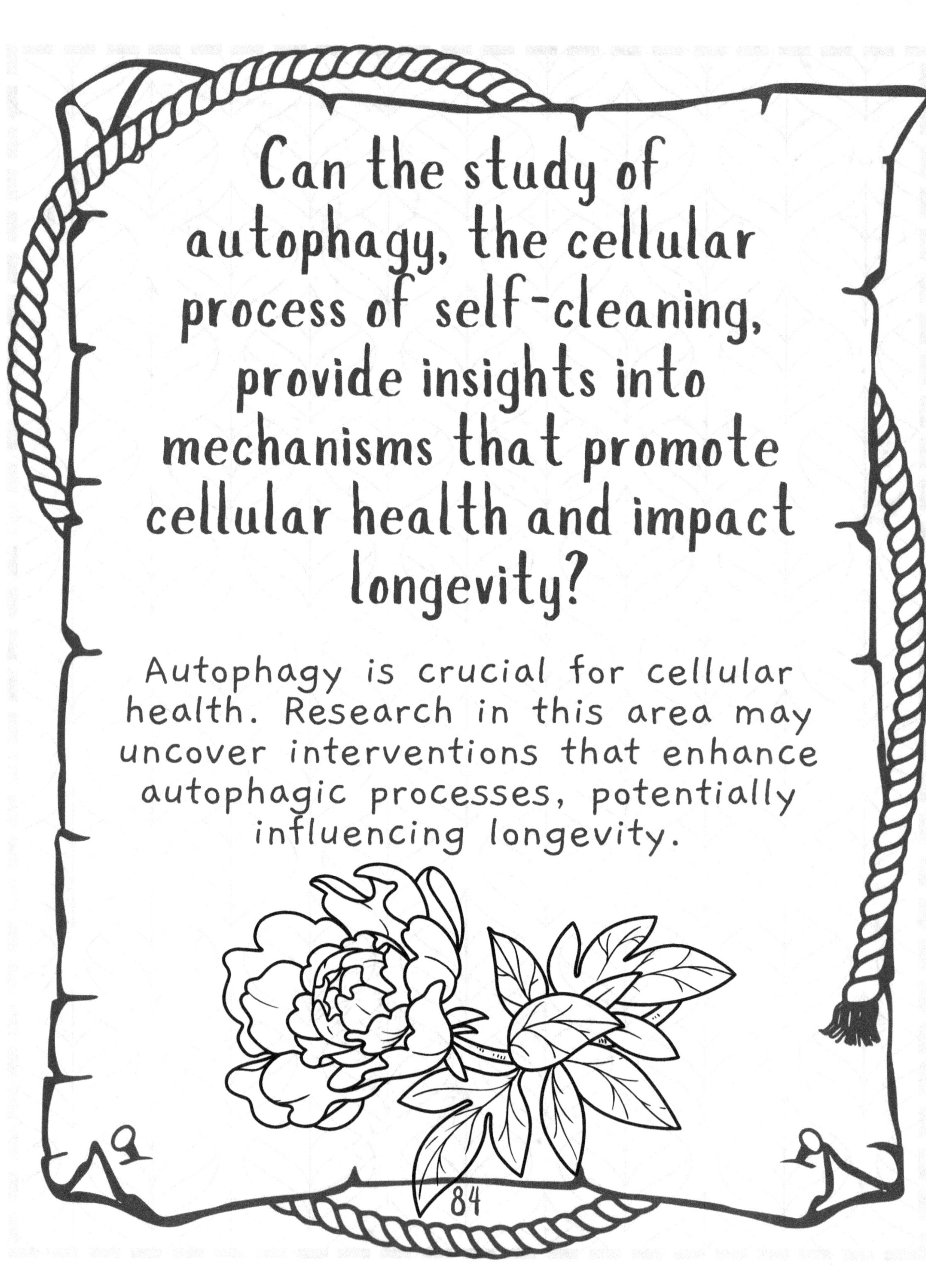

How does the accessibility of green technology and sustainable practices impact environmental health and, consequently, public health and longevity?

Access to green technology and sustainable practices can positively impact environmental health, contributing to public health and potentially influencing longevity.

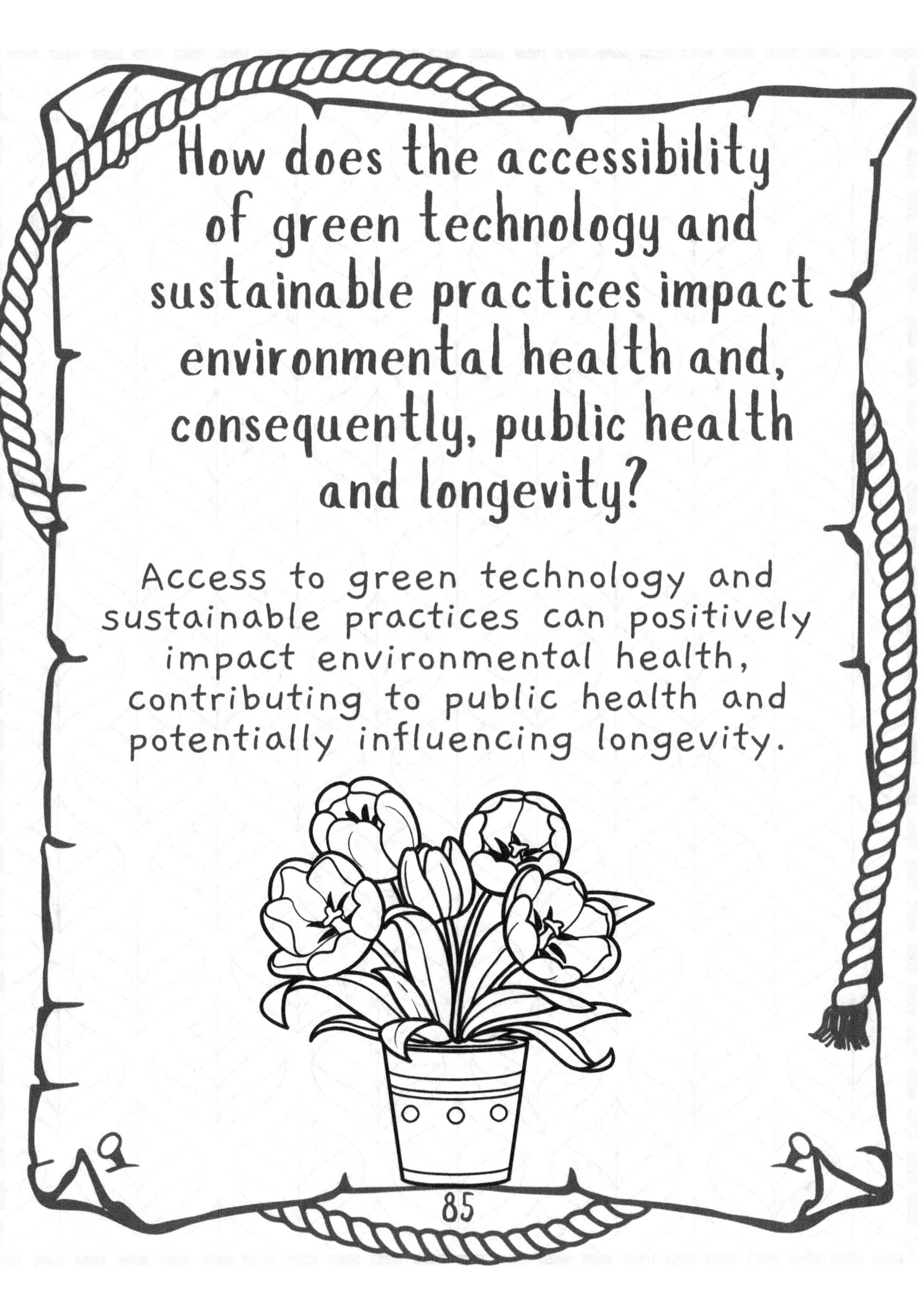

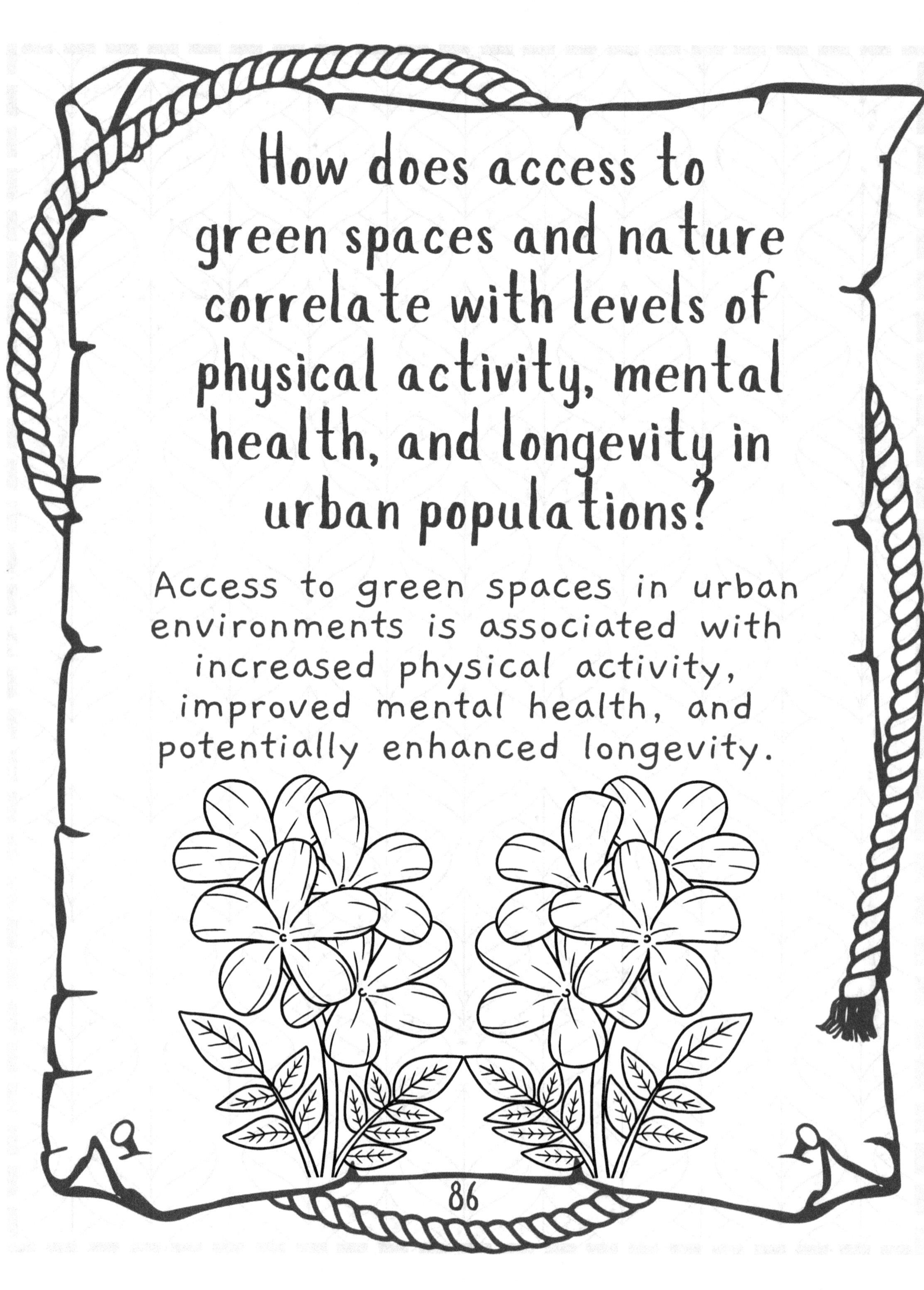

How does access to green spaces and nature correlate with levels of physical activity, mental health, and longevity in urban populations?

Access to green spaces in urban environments is associated with increased physical activity, improved mental health, and potentially enhanced longevity.

Can the integration of artificial intelligence in healthcare systems enhance preventive measures, early detection, and personalized interventions, potentially impacting longevity?

AI applications in healthcare can enhance preventive measures, enable early disease detection, and offer personalized interventions, potentially contributing to increased longevity.

How do societal perceptions of aging impact research funding and prioritization in the field of longevity studies?

Societal attitudes toward aging influence research priorities and funding allocations, shaping the direction of longevity studies and interventions.

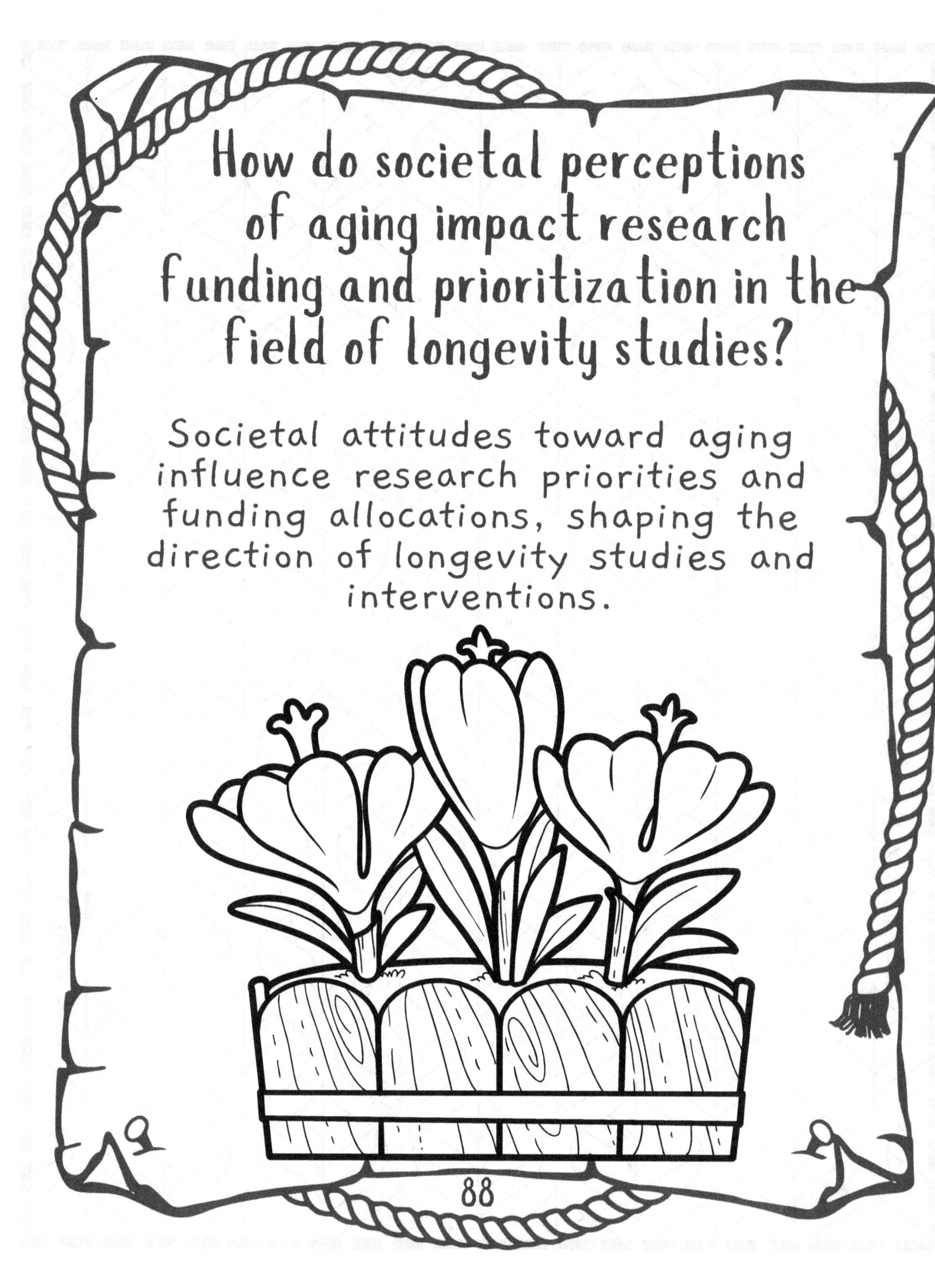

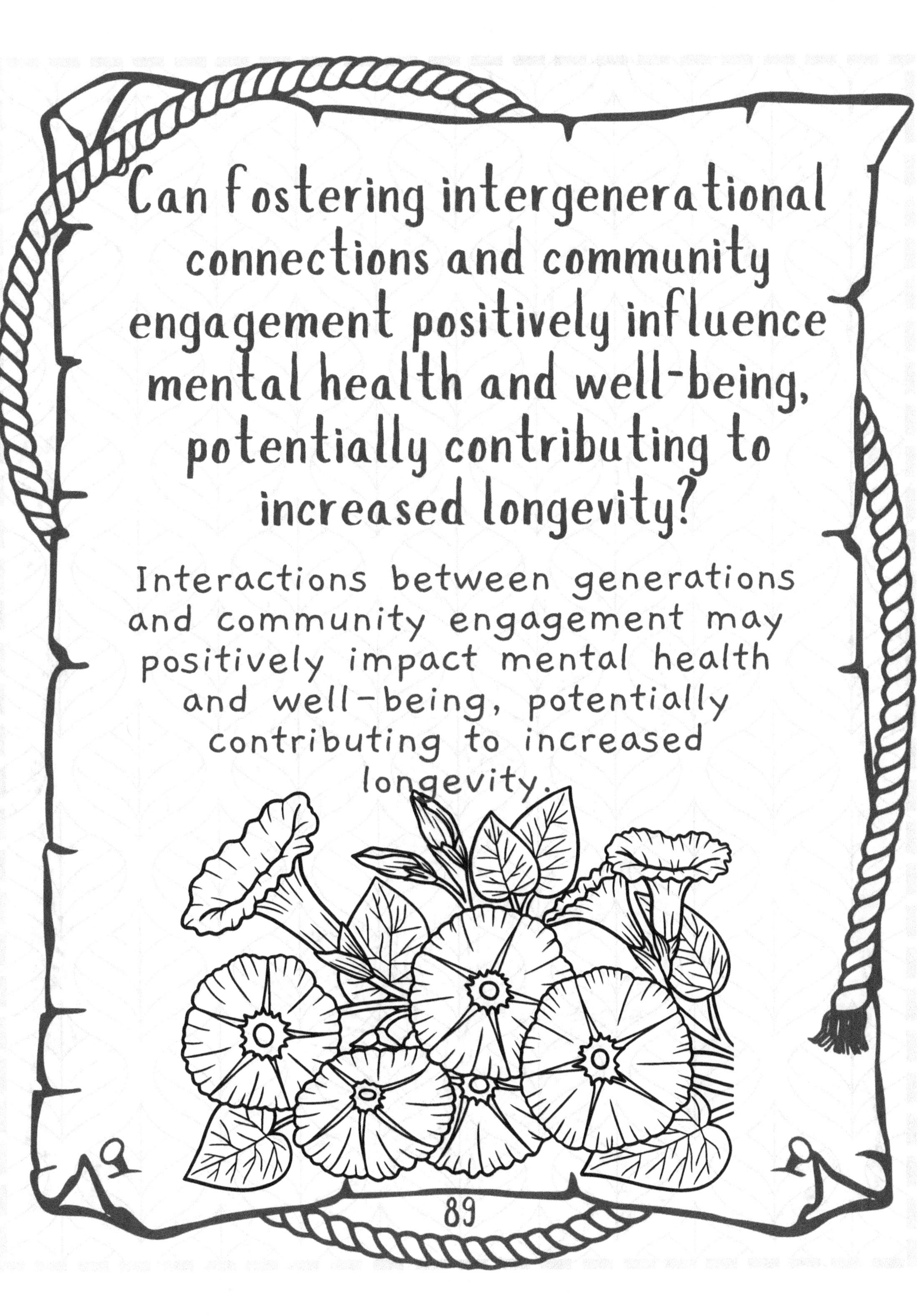

Can fostering intergenerational connections and community engagement positively influence mental health and well-being, potentially contributing to increased longevity?

Interactions between generations and community engagement may positively impact mental health and well-being, potentially contributing to increased longevity.

How does the role of cultural and social traditions in end-of-life care influence perceptions of aging and impact the overall experience of longevity?

Cultural and social traditions in end-of-life care shape perceptions of aging and influence the overall experience of longevity, considering not only lifespan but also the quality of life in later stages.

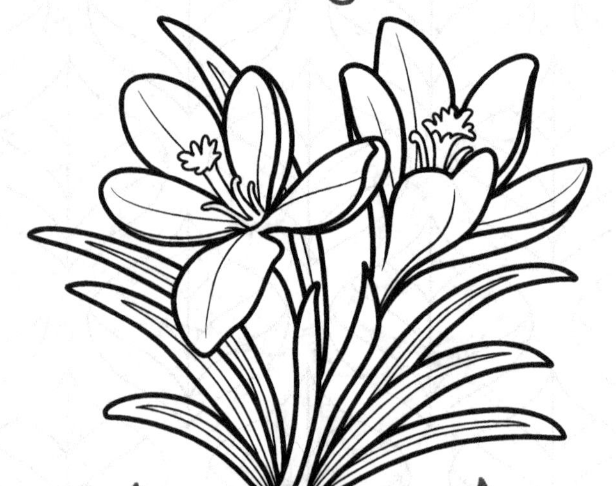

Can advancements in wearable biosensors and continuous health monitoring lead to early detection of age-related health issues, enabling timely interventions for improved longevity?

Wearable biosensors and continuous health monitoring may enable early detection of health issues, allowing for timely interventions that could positively impact longevity outcomes.

How do socioeconomic and cultural factors influence dietary choices and nutrition-related health outcomes, potentially affecting longevity in diverse populations?

Socioeconomic and cultural factors play a significant role in dietary choices, impacting nutrition-related health outcomes and potentially influencing longevity in diverse populations.

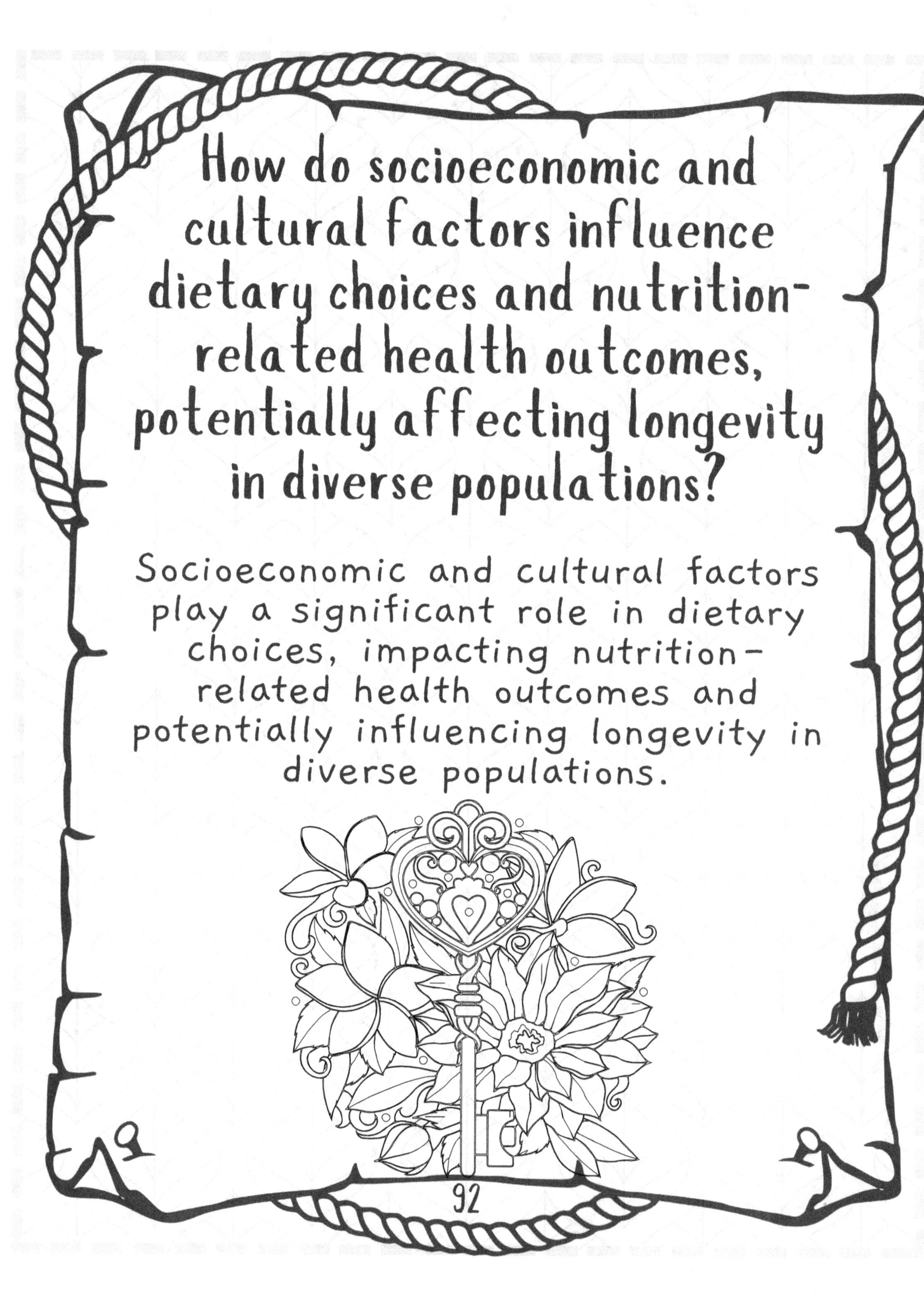

Can the study of non-coding RNAs provide insights into gene regulation and molecular processes that influence the aging process and longevity?

Non-coding RNAs play a role in gene regulation. Studying these molecules may provide insights into molecular processes influencing the aging process and longevity.

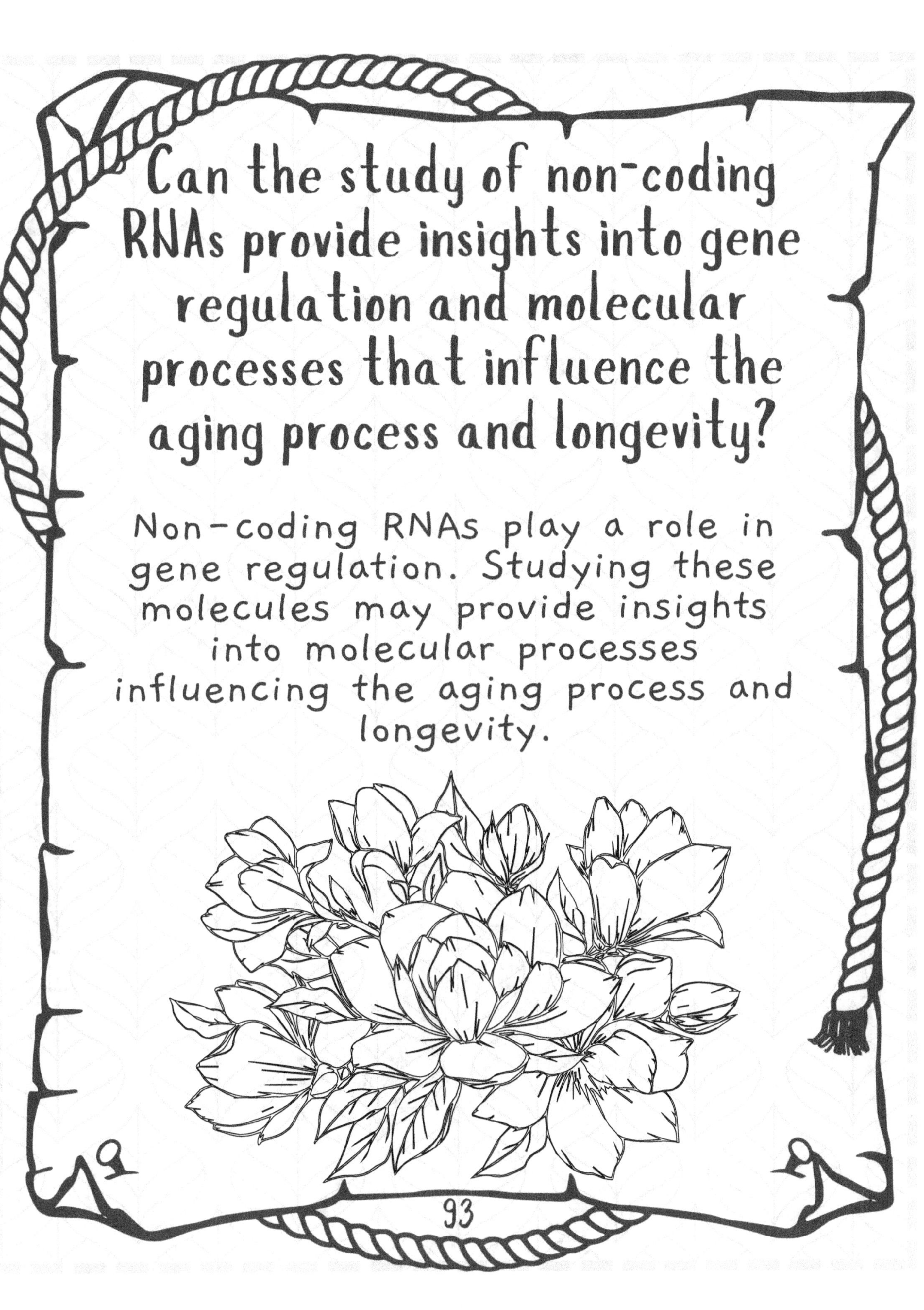

How does the quality of primary and preventive healthcare impact health outcomes and longevity in different healthcare systems globally?

The quality of primary and preventive healthcare is crucial for health outcomes and longevity. Disparities in healthcare systems can impact longevity outcomes globally.

Can mindfulness-based interventions and practices positively impact stress management and mental resilience, potentially influencing longevity outcomes?

Mindfulness-based interventions may contribute to stress management and mental resilience, potentially impacting longevity outcomes by promoting overall well-being.

How does the integration of nutritional education in school curricula influence long-term dietary habits and potentially impact longevity in future generations?

Nutritional education in schools can influence long-term dietary habits, potentially impacting the health and longevity of future generations.

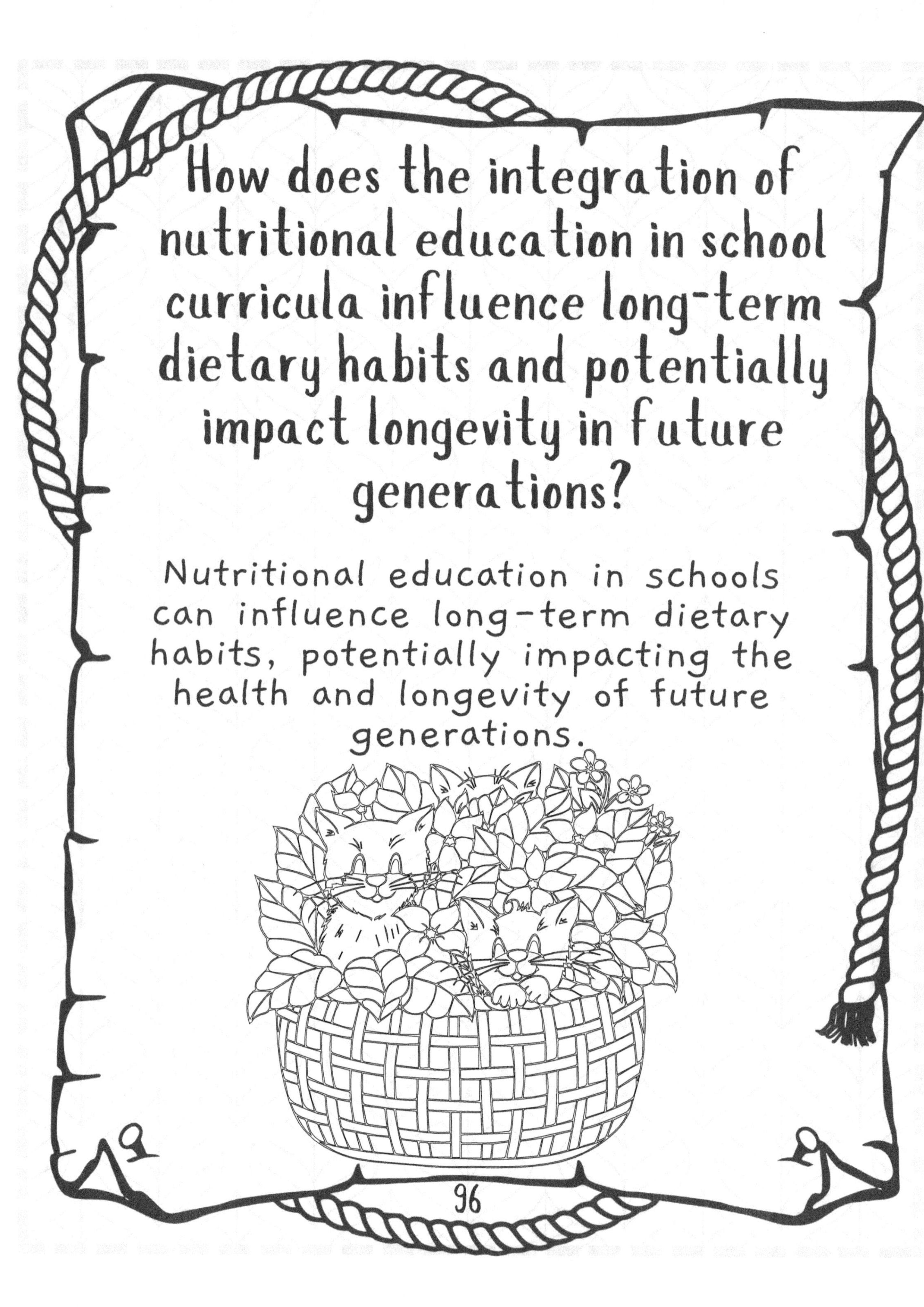

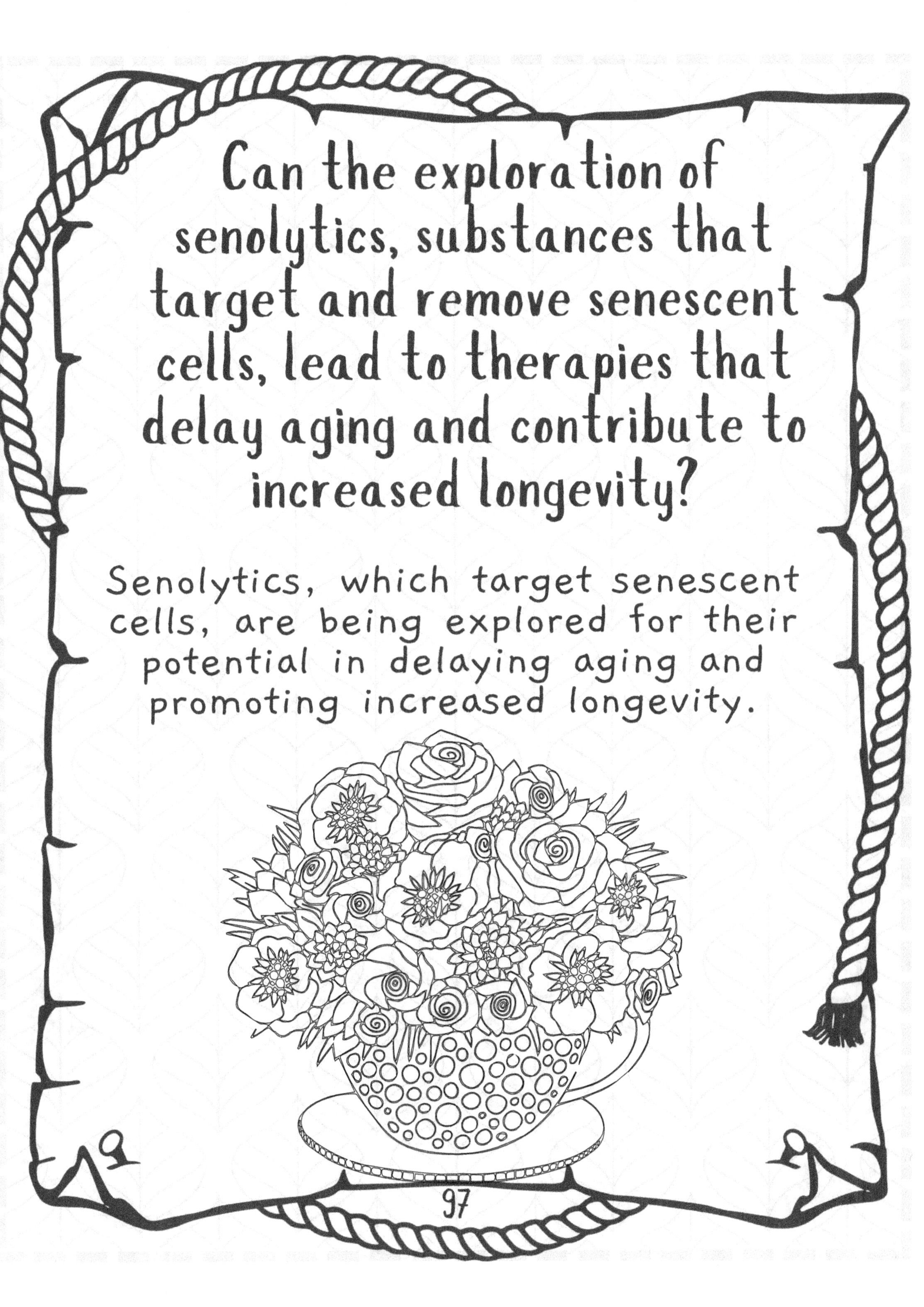

Can the exploration of senolytics, substances that target and remove senescent cells, lead to therapies that delay aging and contribute to increased longevity?

Senolytics, which target senescent cells, are being explored for their potential in delaying aging and promoting increased longevity.

How do government policies related to environmental conservation and pollution control impact public health and longevity on a national scale?

Government policies on environmental conservation and pollution control have implications for public health, potentially influencing longevity outcomes on a national scale.

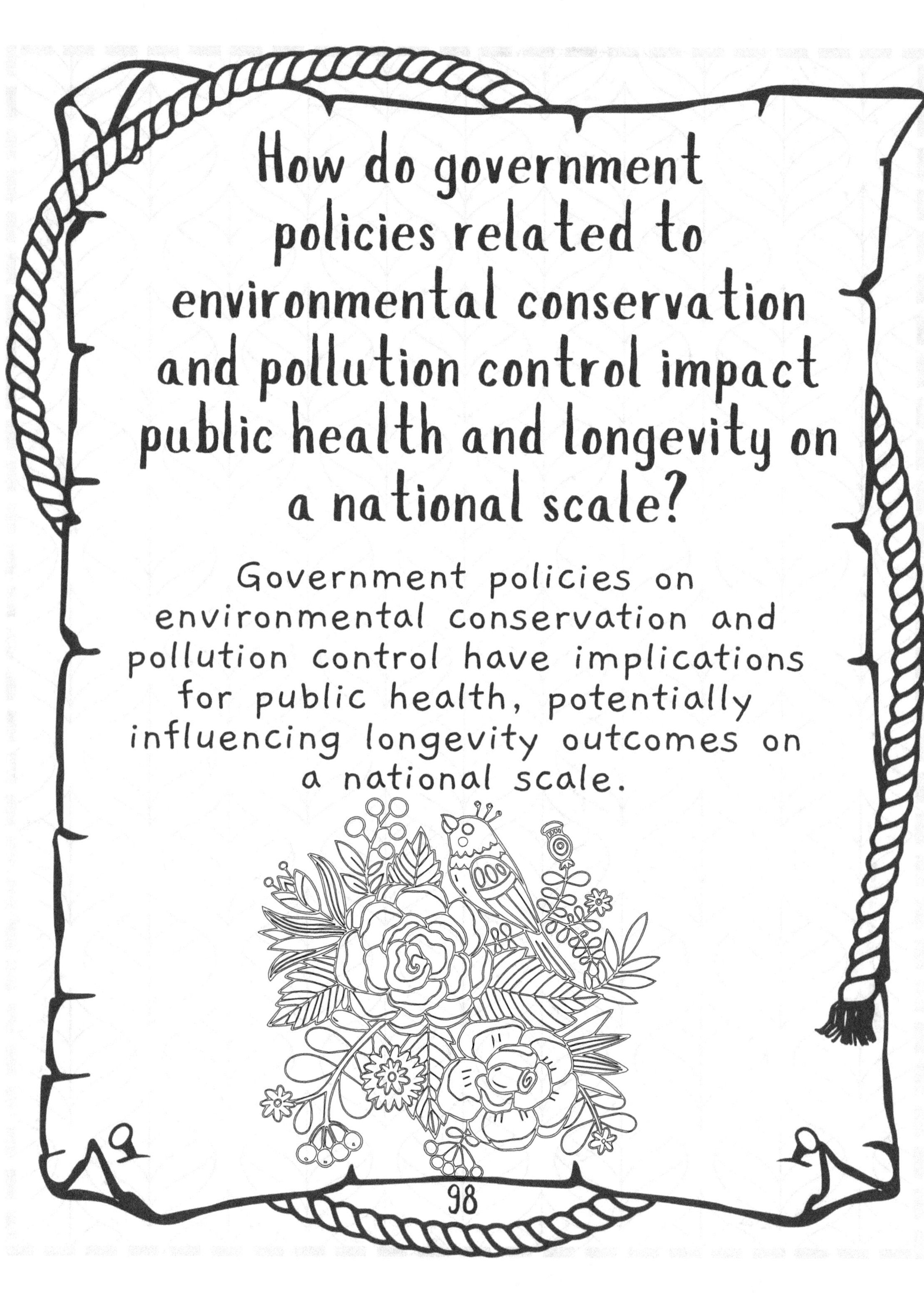

Can the study of social determinants of health provide insights into the root causes of health disparities and inform strategies for improving overall longevity?

Understanding social determinants of health helps identify root causes of disparities, informing strategies to improve overall longevity by addressing systemic factors.

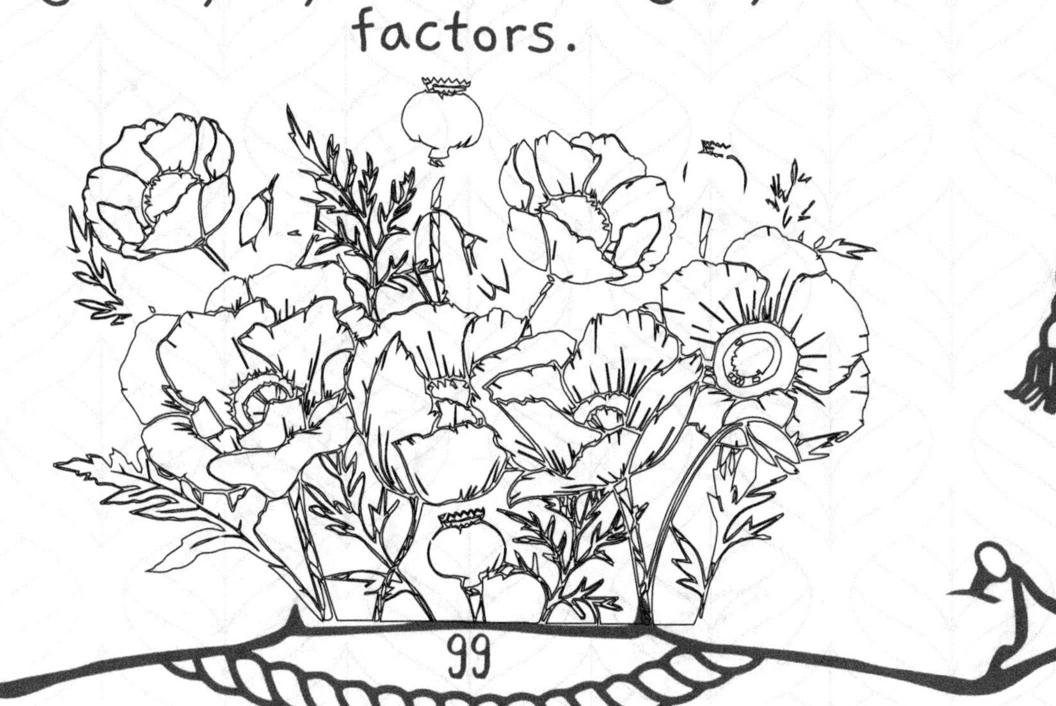

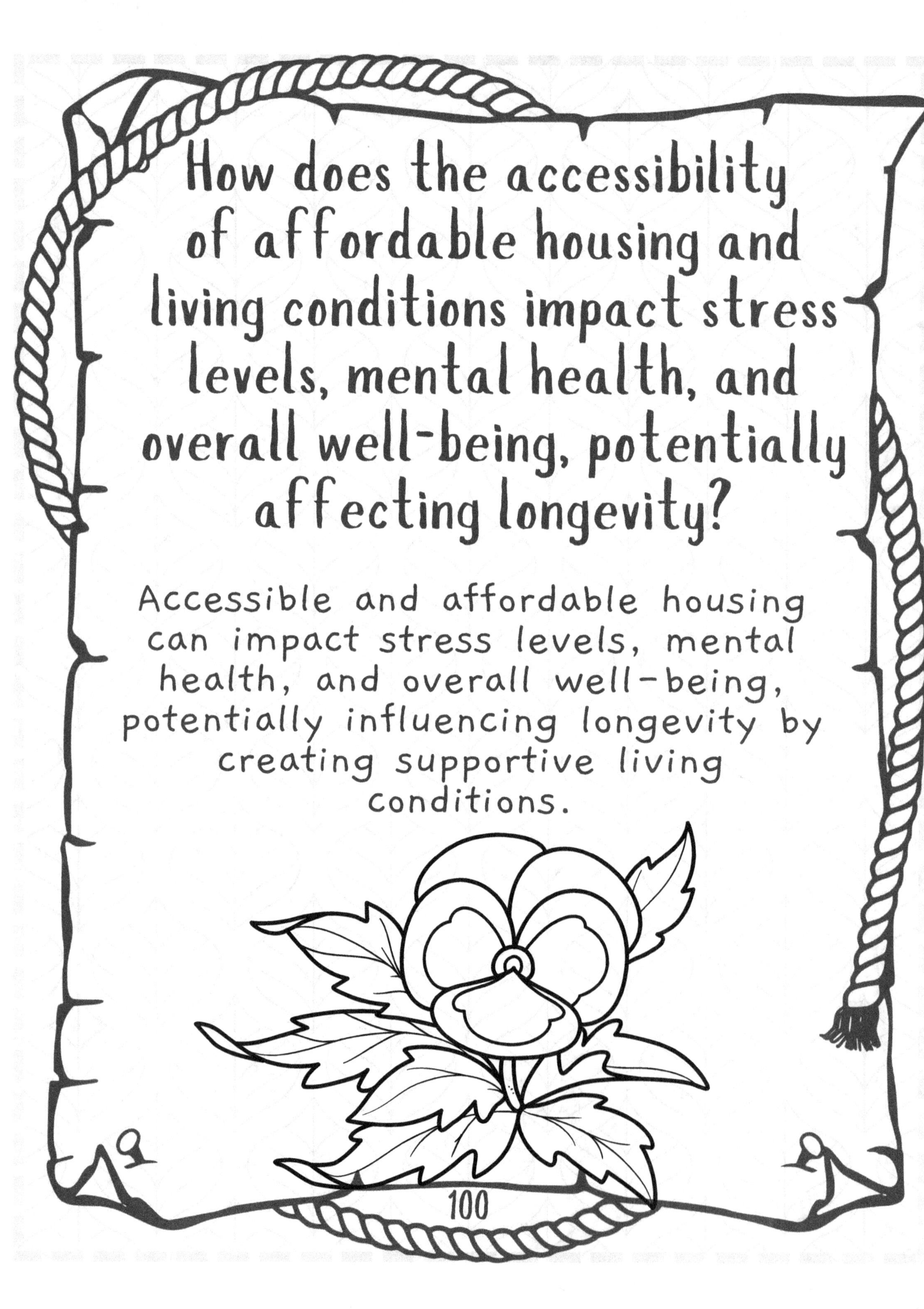

How does the accessibility of affordable housing and living conditions impact stress levels, mental health, and overall well-being, potentially affecting longevity?

Accessible and affordable housing can impact stress levels, mental health, and overall well-being, potentially influencing longevity by creating supportive living conditions.

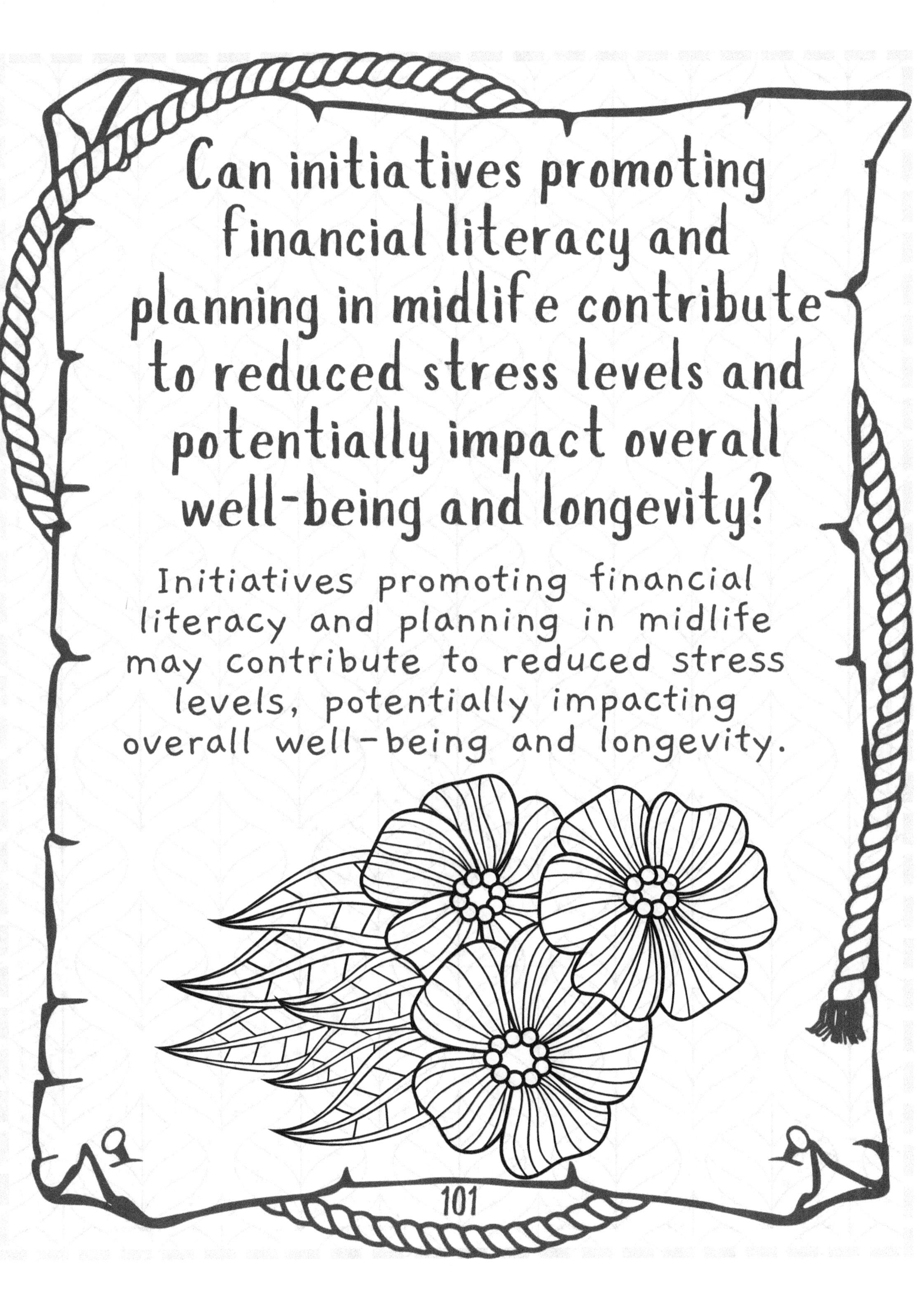

Can initiatives promoting financial literacy and planning in midlife contribute to reduced stress levels and potentially impact overall well-being and longevity?

Initiatives promoting financial literacy and planning in midlife may contribute to reduced stress levels, potentially impacting overall well-being and longevity.

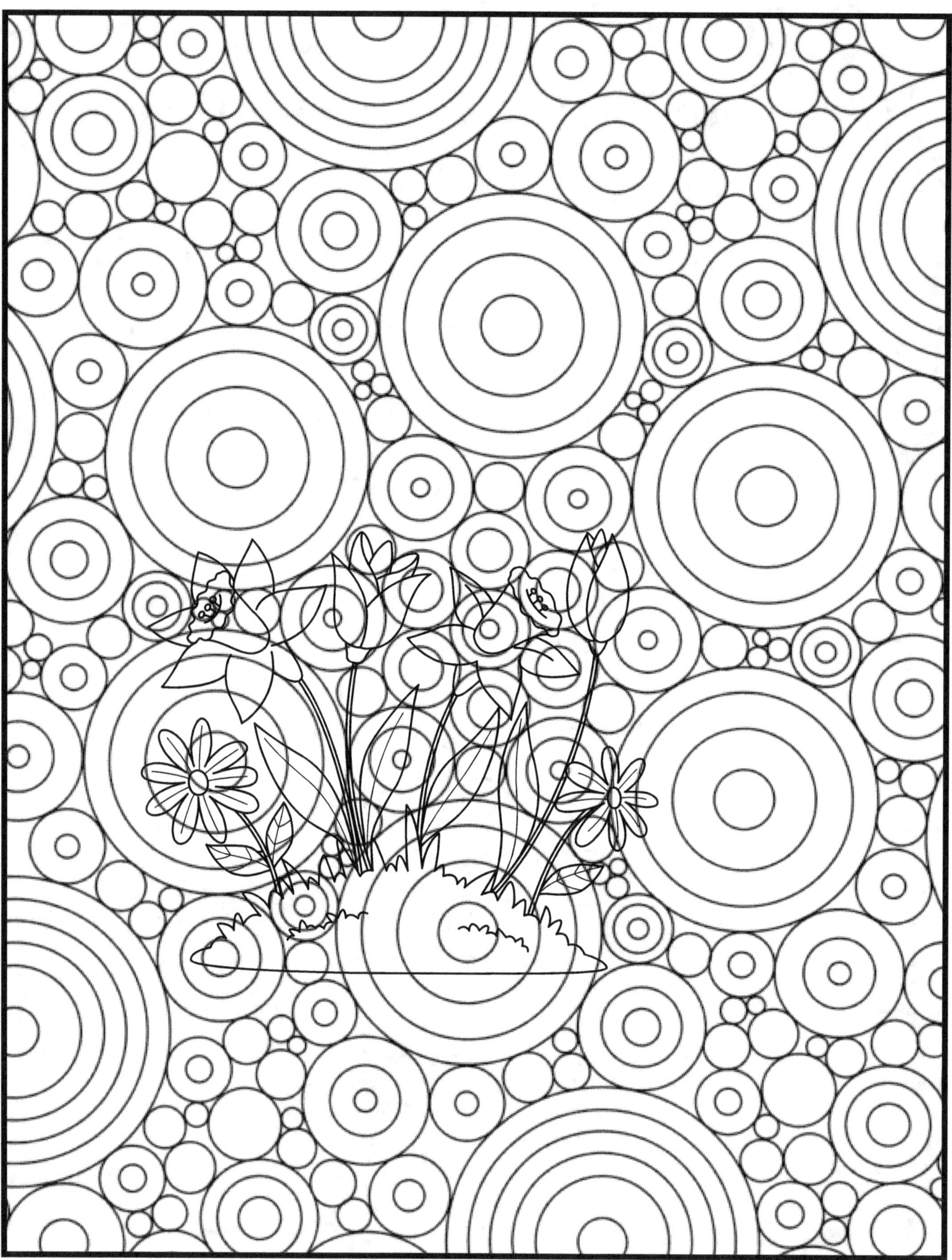